One Man's Journey
Through
Prostate Cancer

BUDD NIELSEN

ISBN 978-1-0980-1771-2 (paperback)
ISBN 978-1-0980-1772-9 (digital)

Christian Faith Publishing, Inc.
832 Park Avenue
Meadville, PA 16335
www.christianfaithpublishing.com

Printed in the United States of America

INTRODUCTION

As you read through my words within this book, I'll be sharing with you a lengthy journey I went on, which started, believe it or not, on a beautiful sunny and pleasant day. My journey began that fateful day the moment I placed the phone to my ear to answer an incoming call. The conversation started obviously with me saying hello and immediately went downhill from there, and I mean downhill fast, like off-the-edge-of-a-cliff fast. The call regrettably was from Doctor Cowan, my urologist, who had been seeing me for many years. His reason for calling, unfortunately, was to inform me that my test results came back from the pathology lab and that those results showed I was indeed clinically diagnosed with cancer. The dreadful darkness begins.

The instant his words left the phone and filtered into my ears, my whole body sank. It was like a dark whirlwind surrounded my body and was pulling the life out. My heart began to speed up, and I began to feel it pounding within my chest. My lungs froze, I couldn't breathe, I also felt a pounding pressure coursing in my ears, and the back of my neck was heating up. My mind couldn't believe what it was hearing. I swear my heart was bursting from fear. At that moment, the word "cancer" became real to me. I felt a cold wind sweep through my mind as it began to spin, as if I was physically dizzy. My mind was petrified. My whole body became weak, and at that moment in time, "Budd's earth stood still." Needless to say, my entire life's perspective was jumbled in just one short second of time.

Very few things in this world will compare to all the different feelings racing through your mind and body at a time like this.

Example: when I was twenty-six, I lived in the intercity, and as I was walking home alone late one evening, a man approached me quite innocently and then abruptly grabbed me, placed a knife to my throat, and robbed me of what I had right there on the city sidewalk. Scary situation. At the time, that was quite horrifying, and I will never forget it, but this one tiny phone call surpassed even that. If you have experienced one of these shocking phone calls, or perhaps you were sitting with your doc when you received the horrible news, believe me when I say you are not alone, I know the pain of what you are going through.

I'm trusting that, by sharing my journey of prostate cancer and all the ups and downs associated with it, it may help ease the substantial burden you or someone you know will be carrying right now as they start their own journey. I'm not a highly educated person, so my choice of words will be in everyday terms, and my hopes are to help you understand some of the difficulties you might encounter (because, my friend, there are many) and to offer some insight to you about the upcoming events plus some supportive understandings into all the little items I found out solely on my own, during my journey—the type of items doctors just don't have the time to sit down with you, hold your hand, and walk you through.

My hope is these insights might prove helpful to you and your family because your family will also be significantly affected. I read many books about prostate cancer written by many different physicians, and they were all filled with insight and knowledge about this subject. Their books helped me greatly and contained many facts, medical terms, physicians' truths, and very helpful information. However, this book is written by a regular guy who speaks in layman's terms and sees through your eyes. I hope my explanation is easy to understand and will calm some of your fears about what to expect and how to prepare yourself for your journey.

Family and Friends.

To begin with, let's start off with a little insight into the "life of Budd." This way, you will get to know the writer of the book a little better before reading on. I was born and raised in Denver, Colorado, a beautiful town in a beautiful state. I'm a second-generation Colorado native, which makes me a bit of a rarity in today's world. I was brought up in a great family with Danish roots. My grandfather was born and raised in Copenhagen, Denmark, and came to the good old United States of America quite unintentionally. He was a sea captain of a supply vessel headed for Liverpool, and while at sea, his ship was chased down and torpedoed by a German U-boat. A day later, he and a few of his crewmembers were rescued from the ocean waves by a passenger ship bound for New York City in the good old USA. The passenger ship obviously had to continue its route and took the rescued sailors with them to America. He liked the states so much he never left. Ended up in Colorado, found a wife, started a new life, and had a baby boy—my father. My grandfather and my father were typical strong Norwegians with wonderful names. My grandfather, Carl Wilhelm Julius Nielsen; my father's name, Odin Thor Nielsen. If you know anything about Viking or Norse mythology and perhaps a few certain aspects of their way of life, you can be certain that the colorful characteristics of the Norsemen presented themselves in both men. My grandfather was quite an energetic character. He raised my father well, and both men, to me, were heroes in every sense of the word.

My dad was a clever man, and over his life span, he literally went from rags to riches. My father started working for his father in a small home repair business, and together, they grew it into a very good construction company. Both my parents (although quite young) lived through and survived the Great Depression. My father taught me many valuable lessons on life. His specialty, relationships, and the family construction business—the art of lath and plastering, installing metal studs, the exterior stucco trade and, later, the fire-proofing of steel I-beams in commercial buildings. He educated me on how to run a business and, more importantly, how to manage money. He also taught me to take care of my mind, body, and spirit. A few valuable lessons from Mr. Odin Thor included: to eat healthy nourishing food but in moderation; exercise your body; expand your mind every day; and to never stop learning. Never stop learning is important—whether it is a minor item or a large thing, learn something each day, even if it was a mistake you made, learn something from it. They were both very positive men.

I grew up in a "man's world," my father's world. He was a strong man, both physically and mentally. My grandfather retired, and my father ruled the business for many years, and when you worked at my dad's company, you did what you were told or you would soon be looking for work elsewhere. It wasn't because my dad was a mean old man. On the contrary, he was good-hearted man, but he knew the dynamics of business and how to efficiently run one. After the workday was over, he could throw down a mug of beer, tell a few tall tales, and make his men laugh. He was such a cool guy, honest and hardworking, someone to look up to, and people just seemed to want to be around him. However, when at work or on the jobsite, no beer of course, just hard work and getting back to efficient business.

I started working for my dad at a very early age, the same as he did with his father. When I was a young boy and we had the "three-month" summer vacation period from school, my father would take me to work with him. He'd grab the collar of my shirt with one hand and the edge of my belt with the other and toss me up into his truck. It was great. I loved it, and of course, as a little kid, it all seemed like fun and games to me. At work, my father showed me how to do specific tasks: what was right, what was wrong, and the reasons behind it all. I really liked watching all the machinery working and especially all the loud and various noises the machines would bellow out plus all the big company trucks groaning under their heavy weighted loads as they passed by with a cloud of dust billowing up behind the rear tires. There were many workers doing various tasks, transporting different tools around the site as they went about their profession. Even though I was a kid, I marveled at the diversity and transformation of the jobsite and how the new building would begin to take shape as it slowly grew out of the ground.

My favorite place to watch all the happenings around the jobsite was from the top of the giant sand pile the workers kept by the cement mixers. High on top of that sand pile, it felt like a pretty safe place for a little kid to be. I was out of the way, and it provided good views of most of the site. Today, with all the safety issues, the insurance policies and OSHA regulations, there's no way a kid would be allowed to do what I did—and with good reason. However, I did it and had fun too. I was blessed to grow up and work in the construction field with my dad and in the same company my grandfather created.

After graduating high school, I worked full-time in the family's company. Just like the other employees that worked for my dad, he was my boss and my friend. It took a few years of hands on work on many different job sites, but I learned a tremendous amount about the job site environments. My father pulled me aside one day and looked me straight in the eye and said, "Son, I'll send you to college if you want to go, but if not, you can come into and be a part of the family business, not just an employee anymore, but part of the office and help run the business alongside me." He said the choice was mine to make. Even though my father was a giant of a man, when he looked me straight in the eye that faithful day, I didn't see a giant, I saw a broken heart if I chose college and didn't follow in his footsteps and go full time into the office as he did with his father. You know, I really didn't want to go to college; high school was difficult enough for me. He and his work were all I knew from a very early age. Two of my friends were already in a college, and a couple of my friends went into the military, but I wanted to be with my dad just like when I was a little boy and he would toss me up into his truck. I'll tell you a little secret: even though my father said it was my choice to make, there really wasn't any choice. I wanted to be there alongside my dad, hands down, no alternative, no backup plan.

When I started working in my father's business on the construction sites, like most employees, I started at the bottom of the ladder. I swept floors, pushed untold numbers of wheelbarrows filled with trash, and cleaned up the construction debris left by the men working on the site. I worked alongside all these men, but because I was young, the older men appeared strong and large in stature, like football players. These workers would carry 100-pound bags of cement to the mixing machines while others shoveled in the sand from the sand piles to mix with the cement. Others installed 14-gauge red steel studs straight and plumb while others welded those studs into their permanent place to make the exterior walls, windows, and door openings. The guys all had a dozen pounds of tools sticking out of tool bags/belts strapped to their waist as they worked all day. This type of environment made a man out of you pretty quick, plus it always seemed as if every guy wanted to prove his "manhood" was superior to the next. Quick witted words, lots of puns, many jokes, and cigarettes were exchanged constantly, and most of the time, it was just loud and jovial. However, occasionally, the words were not so jovial, and the situation quickly turned and the wrong buttons were now being pushed. The joking turned into loud harsh words and then into a shoving match, and of course then the fisticuffs happened, and other guys would be pulling the two men apart and trying to cool off the situation. After which, it was back to work as normal.

I must say, I truly enjoyed working in the family business. My parents worked as a team and were very good at running the business; my father ran all the business logistics, and my mother kept the books, did the banking, and prepared the payroll. Mom and Dad worked side by side, and to me, it seemed like they did this for a hundred years because that was all I knew. They set a fine example of working together, building a business, raising their children, and maintaining a true love story that started when they were both young and growing up in the same school and it just never ended. As the years clocked by, I became more involved with the logistics of running the business. Working side by side with my mom and dad was a great experience; we made a great team and always worked as one mind. Many more years passed, and my father wanted to retire just as his father did. So I took over the company and eventually found myself becoming the same man as my father, which I am proud of. I would regularly hear someone say to me, "You sound just like your old man." I knew occasionally, not often, but sometimes, when those words were spoken to me and the person who said them really meant it as a dishonor toward me or my dad; however, those few words have always been and will forever be a great compliment to me! Whenever I hear those words, no matter how they are spoken, you'll see a cat-like grin appear on my face.

Throughout my life, I have always been interested in how things work. I would tear something apart so I can learn how it works. Learning is the way to keep your mind active, and my dad tried to learn something new every day. I really admired that quality in him. My father took a small business and made into a very productive company. He took chances. He learned new things like how to refine the art of ornamental plastering. He learned how to be a good employer and how to get along with others in the business community, which meant when we would acquire a job, our company's name, "Nielsen," defined professionalism and quality. I continued his example by learning and expanding my mind. It had been fairly easy to do because I had such a great role model. I started to realize how important some of those lessons my dad taught me would prove useful during the upcoming cancer journey.

Cancer is such a dreadful word and comes most often with dreadful fear attached. Over my lifespan, I have watched multiple family members plus a few close friends pass away from various different forms and grades of cancer. Here are few: My grandmother Charlotte, my Aunt Joyce, Uncle Gene, Uncle Donald, cousin Dennis, brother-in-law Gus, my good friend "California Paul," my beautiful sister Peggy, and absolutely the most painful was my amazing father Odin Thor Nielsen.

Peggy, my sister, God bless her soul, was diagnosed with stage 4 brain cancer. The tumor in her brain was spreading like an unchecked fibrous weed and embedding itself within the crevices of her brain. A very ugly form of cancer, and unfortunately, there were no procedures to stop this particular form of cancer. We all painfully watched over a twelve-month period as my sister went from a happy blond-haired healthy and active woman with two children to a small, fragile form of a woman hidden under the blankets on a bed inside the hospice facility where the end of her life played out. The very same hospice facility where, many years later, my family gathered and watched as Odin Thor's fate played out, also after a deadly cancer diagnosis. I dearly miss every family member and friend that we have lost because of that dreadful word.

A word about my friend, "California Paul."

Listen to this little story about Paul, a very nice guy who I met in Northern California, way up north, near the Oregon border. He "was" a fun guy—tall, thin, hippy-length long hair, and a beard. He would have fit right in with ZZ TOP. Anyhow, Mr. Paul, myself, and a few other buddies volunteered to work together for several months to build geodesic domes off the grid and high up in the backwoods of California. (No, we were not hidden militia; we were hippy dudes doing a good deed). A key word for Paul—"was." Paul had been diagnosed with prostate cancer. It so happened that, at the time of his diagnosis, we were all small-time environmentalists, recyclers, and a bunch of self-proclaimed long-haired tree-huggers. We took lots of vitamins and mineral supplements, ate organic food, and stayed away from fried and fast food. We didn't add any MSG to our diets. We ate backwoods honey that drenched our homemade granola bars containing various nuts and fruits; we even made our own beef jerky from squirrel and deer meat plus (everyone's favorite) a tasty homemade treat called fruit leather. But for me, those granola bars we made were my all-time favorite. We were into natural foods and, of course, natural healing, taking care of ailments with natural remedies. For the most part, I still feel that way even today, and all the health stuff we were doing usually worked out reasonably well. However, I have come to realize that some things in this world, and in our lives, will take more help than we ourselves and nature can supply. Nature is great, but some personal battles our bodies will be confronted with need the newest technologies, the latest innovations, and doctors with the brightest minds to beat the odds and enable us to win those battles that confront us.

Back to my friend Paul. After the prostate cancer diagnosis, he did what he could to wage a fighting battle against it, and I'm proud to say he did his best. I must admit, it even looked like he might be winning his battle. He tried all the normal things one would do at such a time when they find themselves in such a trial. He tried all the good and natural remedies. He ate a healthy diet and tried many self-remedies. He stayed fit, exercised, and endlessly searched

the internet to find any late-breaking news of some new herbal prostate mixture to help combat this heart-breaking disease. He searched
for any news regarding antioxidants, which are amazing substances
that actively hunt down any free radicals within the human body
and tries to eradicate them. Paul increased his daily intake of the
good stuff like tofu, soy milk, fruits, lots of grapes, raw almonds,
vegetables, even alfalfa. Paul ate fresh cooked tomatoes by the dozen
and consumed lots of garlic. He used lots of extra-virgin olive oil
and a lot of Omega-3 fatty acids from the town store we would visit
every couple of weeks plus what he got from all the fish we would
take out of the river. He consumed ground flaxseed, which is very
high in Alpha-linolenic acid (I should do more studying on flaxseed
because it needs to be in powder form, not whole flaxseed). Paul got
plenty of herbs and anything else that he thought would help him.
He ate all the antioxidants, vitamins, and good foods for energy that
our human earth suits really need as we live on this third rock from
the sun. We were tree-hugging naturalists and made fresh fruit juice
from a variety of fruits, even vegetable juice from all those cooked
tomatoes mixed up in a blender with spinach and celery. The vegetable juice mix was just like V8. I must admit, it seemed to be a very
healthy way to live and extremely helpful for the nourishment of our
bodies. Another lesson from my dad.

But here is the dark side to this tale. Within Paul's body was
a silent deadly monster—a monster that was determined to take
over his body and then take over his life. Now, being totally honest,
while we were living this healthy lifestyle, we were able to control the
majority of ailments. This time, unfortunately, Paul's mountain was
too high and too steep for him to climb. Paul passed away twelve
years after his diagnosis of prostate cancer. This is no joke; he was
on my mind for some reason one month before I myself received
the horrible phone call from my doctor who informed me that I was
diagnosed with the same ugly monster as Paul was. Thank God for
my urologist, Dr. Cowan, for his knowledge, his wisdom, and years
of education. All these combined together and helped me in having
an early cure. I wish my buddy Paul would have done more research
before he decided to go down the road he chose; however, that's

hindsight, but hindsight did help me, plus it is easy to say now what he should have done back then. Kinda like being a Monday morning armchair quarterback. However, I do remember reading somewhere that close to 200,000 cases of prostate cancer are discovered each year and approximately 10 percent actually die of it. That bit of news is old news now, so the numbers are most likely slightly up from those.

CHAPTER 1

Prostate Health—before the diagnosis

I have to say now that, in reality, years before my doctor's horrifying phone call is when my cancer journey actually began. It was during one of my normal physical visits with my main doctor—my general practitioner. He suggested it would be a good idea (at my young age, ha-ha!) to visit a good urologist. Strange how things materialize, because I just happened to know a very good urologist. You see, six years earlier, my wife and I went through a lengthy and definitely very difficult journey through infertility. Throughout that difficult time in our lives, one doctor (Cowan) out of the many doctors we visited with was part of a cool group of physicians called Urology Associates.

Later that day, when I returned home from my general practitioner physical, I explained to my wife what he suggested I do (have the urologist visit). She was hot on the trail. She called Urology Associates and set up my first visit. At this visit, I was reintroduced to Dr. Cowan. The visit went well. Dr. Cowan did all of the usual things, including the dreaded glove test. The doctor visited with me and took some notes. Everything turned out good enough, and I was set up for my second appointment six months in the future, and he would like to see me on a continual basis of every six months thereafter (something all men some do). At my second appointment, Dr.

Cowan performed his normal exam and looked over his previous notes plus the notes he had from my general physician who sent me to him in the first place. He said, in his opinion, he felt that I had a "slightly" enlarged prostate gland but nothing out of the normal for my age and no red flags. From what the notes indicated from our first visit to what he was now noticing, there was nothing alarming or out of the ordinary. Just a slightly enlarged prostate and enlarging is a normal occurring performance of the prostate gland. I think it was on my fourth visit to him which would be a timeline of two years of accumulated visits. He said that he thought it would be prudent to have some outside testing done. This was where a few more small pieces of the puzzle first began to come together. One of the outside tests he wanted to do was a prostatic specific antigen test (PSA test). To explain PSA to you, I'll say it like this: our prostate gland produces what is known as a protein (or antigen), and this protein is labeled as PSA and it's found in our blood, since it's in the blood. When the lab draws a blood sample from you, they can then look for that specific antigen and will measure its level. That definition you just read is extremely simple and is all mine. You should (as with any information in this book) check it out with your doctor or urologist. This is a simple blood test that might perhaps help in detecting the possible presence of prostate cancer, or it may just show the normal effects of getting older. It is important that I explain to you that these PSA test results should not be interpreted as absolute evidence of the presence or absence of this disease regardless of the results. This PSA test number is more like a guideline to use and to help you and your doctor decide which path to take for future health concerns and which steps would be more beneficial for you. They are not a positive note of cancer.

Here's some information for you. Normal PSA levels range from 0.0 to 4.0. The lower the number, obviously the better. However, even a level of a 4.0 may not be a cause for alarm—that's still an acceptable range. Once the PSA levels rise above 4.0, you may start to think about it, and yet, it is still not an alarming level. However, you and your doctor should at least sit up and start to take notice and begin to check into the reason why the level is raising above 4.0.

There are several reasons for an elevated level, and one of those reasons might be—I repeat, might be—an indication of prostate cancer, but it would be way out on the side line at best. The level is one reason why it should be investigated, because this is an issue that should be addressed. Please take it from the one who wrote this book: the sooner you find out why these numbers have their continuous but slow and steady raise and what is causing these issues, the less has to be done to correct it exactly like preventive maintenance on anything, plus, the earlier detected, the high percentage of a healthier future outcome, which makes the odds hugely stacked in your favor. Don't roll the dice on this one, brother!

Since my journey began, I have spoken with many prostate cancer survivors because I wanted and needed to speak with different men that had gone through this. I needed multiple opinions (another lesson I learned from my dad) so I could make an intelligent decision for my own course of action, which is something you should also consider. In all the test case scenarios that I have studied, it seems that the guys with the earliest detections have the brightest outcomes with the fewest problems now and later. The longer you wait, the tighter the hold cancer can get, and the more aggressive it may become. This is important, so take note. Aggressive cancer inside your body is never good. Also important—the longer you wait, the fewer options you might have to combat this enemy. Many of the gentlemen I spoke with are living with everyday problems that they will face for the rest of their lives, including myself. This may affect you for the rest of your life, so it's good to talk to others who have been in this situation and walked this journey. They know the reality of what you're going through and can offer insight.

This is my best advice to every man: Get a good doctor on your side. Go to the appointments to have the dreaded glove test and also get PSA tests done, at the very least, once every year. I went to my doctor and did both—glove and PSA test—every six months. Now get this, because I had frequent visits, my doc was on top of the situation and was able to spot anything that he thought was just a wee bit unusual. These doctors are in their respective professions because they care about people and they want to help you; they want you to have a good prosperous life. Detect it early and eradicate it early as possible. In this situation, you don't want a yellow flag thrown for delay of game.

Some more information for you: Every guy needs to be tested by a urologist and tested early in this game. Most of the studies I have read state that, by age fifty, a man should start having regular yearly checkups. I personally think forty years of age is a good starting point for men to be tested once a year. The reason I say forty is that, right around the age of twenty-eight, our male prostate begins its own little growth program unbeknownst by you and will continue this growth most likely 'til the end of days. Most physicians recommend age fifty, and as with everything, you should always discuss this with your medical provider. But if you are age fifty or older and have never had a urology checkup or PSA testing done, then get off your doctor fearing—and man up! This information I'm telling you is not only for your benefit, brother, but you have to understand, you also have loved ones who love you and are depending on you. You don't want to let them down when a simple visit to the doctor once a year is a proactive step toward taking care of your health, your future, and taking care of your family too. We do maintenance on our cars, why not on our own bodies?

My first PSA test results were in the normal range at 3.0. At this level, there was no need for worry or concern. I felt normal—no pain, no side effects, and there didn't seem to be anything that would set off an alarm or raise a red flag to my doc or myself. However, and this is the kicker, neither one of us knew there may be an ugly monster slipping his dreadful form into that which was not his. I didn't have any of the characteristic early effects which are: an unusually hard-to-start urine flow or the extremely slow and longer lasting flow, bladder infections, urinary tract infections, or kidney problems. Those are signs that are usually associated with an enlarged prostate, so at this time in my journey, I was OK, sort of like running under the radar. Over the next couple of years, each one of my six-month visits to the urologist showed the PSA test results were slightly higher than the one before. It had gone up a split fraction of a point. Just slightly higher, never a huge jump at any one time.

This also is why you personally, not just your doctor, but both of you need to study your PSA test results, because this slow and steady uphill trend is a telling factor. A few more pieces of the puzzle were coming together, and I did not like the picture coming into focus. Fortunately, I started my testing early, and that proved to be incredibly important. Because I did start my doctor visits early and I also started my PSAs early, my doctor had my "baseline" level, which is an excellent benchmark (a great starting point) for any doctor to determine what is normal for their patient, and just as important, you will know what is not normal. So jumping ahead a little, Dr. Cowan had seen me early, he had seen me twice a year over the years, he performed all the normal exams, made many notes, and had a good understanding of my health while in the normal PSA range. So now he was able to see a slow but steady increase in my PSA test scores as each one came back to him. Plus, he was educated on my normal prostate glands size and hardness because he had performed the golden glove test on me each time I visited his office. After adding all this information together from over the years, the signs were not pointing in an encouraging direction; however, they were still in the normal range, so all things considered, it was not a terribly ugly position either.

My doc quizzed me about my "urine flow rate" because one of the biggest side effects of an enlarged prostate is the flow rate of urine. It has a tendency to slow down gradually over time or you can have uncomfortable blocking of the flow or difficulty starting and stopping and also a very slow flow and drips at the end which, unfortunately, ends up in your underwear—just a few wonderful things. A bit more information for you men out there. Please check your own flow rate and take note of the normal rate you have and monitor it over time and make notes of any changes. This is not an easy thing to do because it changes so slowly. If you aren't paying attention, you will not even notice the subtle change. Myself, I didn't notice it at all, but I wasn't checking it either, and of course, no one told me to check it, so I was not even aware of it changing slowly over time. Because the urine flow rate takes place so slowly over a number of years, it won't be too noticeable unless you are actively paying attention. However, if you have some very close and well-meaning friends like I did, they might just tell you, "Dude, you're slow."

Example: Whenever myself, along with my group of close friends, went to our local brew pub for a night out, like we had for years, my buddies unknowingly noticed this little thing for me. They came right out and told me, "Budd, what's up with you, man? Whenever we go to the men's room, you really spend a long time at the urinal."

Of course, I would dismiss their comments by explaining it as, "Hey, bigger pipes take longer to empty." In reality, it did take me a little longer to empty my oil tank than the time it took my friends. Honestly, if it hadn't been for my doctor's questions about my flow rate and also for my well-meaning friends quizzing me on the length of time I was spending at the urinal, I probably wouldn't have been aware that I was indeed slowing down over time. Now that I have mentioned this fact to you, maybe you will take heed of yours also.

Another note to be aware of is the second sign of a troubled prostate gland, which is having trouble at the very beginning when you are trying to start the flow of urine in the first place. You physically feel like you have to go, you have the urge to go, and yet it is a little difficult to get it started. For me I didn't have this second sign. It wasn't difficult for me to start the flow. When I felt the urge and stepped up to the plate, the flow started with ease, but now, I was becoming aware of it being a little slower flow rate. I didn't want to admit it, but the facts were there, right in front of me, almost like if I was holding them in my hand.

"Our prostate gland," as described in Budd words. When our male prostate gland is of normal healthy size, it's approximately the size of a walnut. It should be rather soft, and I would describe it as almost springy to the touch. Also, when it is compared with other organs in the male body, our little gland is quite small. Here's the real issue with our walnut-sized gland; it is basically constructed in the shape of a donut with a donut hole obviously right in the middle. Now, please don't go around telling people that Budd said, "It looks just like a donut." It doesn't actually look like a physical donut such as the ones from Dunkin Donuts. It's more of an egg shape (oval) just like a walnut; however, the urethra tube carrying our urine does travel into the top of our gland, down through the center of the gland, and out the bottom of our gland, and that positioning of the urethra tube running through the center of the gland, is why I used the metaphor of a donut. The tube creates what, you could say, is a wormhole traveling completely through the center of the gland and through entire length of our gland. So for us guys, our exit tube for urine really begins or starts at the base of our bladder and runs downhill to the top of the prostate gland, where this tube then passes right through the center of this donut hole and then obviously out the bottom of the gland and continues downhill toward and through our penis. (This is my layman's terms for describing the urinary tract). As our prostate gland gets larger, the donut hole in the center gets smaller and—that's right, you guessed it—the flow gets restricted and, of course, slows down and may even create a situation where it is possibly harder for a man to start his flow, and get this, at times, it may be difficult to even stop at times without a bunch of drips occurring and coming out later.

Now, if you will, I shall describe it for you in medical terms which is a little longer in description and uses improved words. The whole journey is part of the "male genitourinary system." It starts within the bladder, which is basically the holding tank for our urine. At the very bottom-lower end of the bladder is an area called the trigone, and this is where the bottom of the bladder turns into the urinary exit tube and is called the ureteral orifice; this is also where our tube begins. The tube goes down and through the center of the first set of sphincter muscles, the internal urethral sphincter. After exiting the sphincter, our exit tube at this point is called the prostatic urethra, apparently named such because it runs straight through the center of the prostate gland, which we'll touch on more a little later (no pun intended). The prostatic urethra tube, after passing through the center of the prostate gland and coming out the lower-bottom side of the prostate now runs through the second set of sphincters, the external urethral sphincter, and of course, the name changes again; it is now called the membranous urethra than the bulbous urethra, and finally, the last and longest run is called the pendulous or the penile urethra, naturally named because it now runs down and through the center of the penis and exits through the external urethral opening. It's all the same long tube, but in medical terms, the name of our urethra tube changes due to the area it is traveling through and is associated with.

OK, here's where the problems start. As our male prostate gland begins to enlarge, the little hole in the middle naturally begins to shrink in diameter but very gradually; it's just the way our body works. This gradual shrinking size of the hole which is encircling the urethra tube now has a stranglehold on our little exit tube. This stranglehold is slowly and gradually shutting down the flow of urine which, in turn, causes us to take a little longer to drain our fuel tank. In the very beginning, there's no pain associated with this condition. After a long length of time (multiple years), when this condition gets further along and difficulty of starting a stream and a small amount pain comes, that's when we begin to sit up and take notice. I didn't notice it at all because I had zero pain associated with the slowdown, so to me, all appeared quite normal—no pain, no red flags, no alarms, no worries. It wasn't until after my doc questioned me several different times about my flow rate and my buddies teased me about my urinal time that I began to realize I should be giving this more thought, and it was a good thing I did, so thanks to all of you for bringing it to my attention.

After I'm in heaven and walk through those pearly gates, one of the many questions I will be asking is why in the world did you design this thing in a donut shape? I have a few ideas of my own for a better shape than a donut, but then again, I don't think my ideas will carry much influence with the big guy up there! I can only imagine there is probably an excellent reason for the design, and perhaps it assists with the function of our gland, which is reproduction. The prostate gland adds fluid and mixes that fluid together with the sperm males produce, and all that ends up together in our exit tube. I think that the fluid helps in the flow of sperm and its mobility. Like the oil in our vehicle engines, it helps all the parts work together with less friction and maybe even makes our sperm go further and swim faster. Yeah.

OK, here's a recap of what we have just learned. As the prostate gland increases in size, the small donut hole in the middle does the opposite and decreases in size (diameter). Our exit tube is now beginning to get squeezed smaller and smaller over a longer and longer period of time, which is why the flow slows down. Thankfully, Dr. Cowan knew about the flow rate, and this is surely why he asked me about my own flow. However, he never expanded further to me about the flow rate or even what the flow rate should be like at its normal point. Thinking back, I kind of wish my doc would have asked me to measure and monitor the flow in the beginning so we could have had a guideline or baseline early in the whole process.

At this point, due to my doc asking me and my good friends teasing me, I started to pay attention to the speed of my flow and also the volume of the flow. I'm familiar with the system of hydraulics; there is speed, and there is volume. An example of flow rate would be kind of like a backyard garden hose. If you place a sprinkler on the end of the garden hose, one that produces a nice round spray of water, and turn the water on full force, you would notice the beautiful round full spray of water coming forth. You will notice two things: lots of volume, and lots of speed. As you watch the water spraying out of the sprinkler, you should take note of the speed of the water as it exits the sprinkler and also get a good idea of how far the water is traveling out and away from the sprinkler. This distance of travel now becomes your baseline for all future observations. Once you have observed the water for a minute or so, you would then notice if there is any deviation from this baseline. So now while you're monitoring the waters full flow, grab a pair of pliers and use these pliers to slowly clamp down somewhere in the middle of the water hose. As your hands very slowly squeeze down on the plier handles, you will begin to notice the flow rate of the water is not as forceful or as fast and, consequently, will not spray out as far, nor will it have the volume of water as our baseline once had. Well, this is exactly what is happening inside your body. You may not notice the slowing down of the flow because it happens so gradually; I'm talking like over many years. The pliers, on the other hand, make the garden hose "flow rate" happen quickly and is quite obvious. The flow of water in the garden hose is far greater than our little man hose and much easier to measure. The average household garden hose flow rate is measured in gallons-per-minute (GPM), which is pretty fast. Human males obviously have smaller hoses, and therefore, we have smaller flow rates and can't be measured in GPM's, we are measured in milliliters-per-second (MLPs). The flow of the garden hose is pretty easy to calculate. Get a five-gallon bucket, a stopwatch, and no nozzles on the end of the garden hose—just free flow. Start the watch as soon as you start filling the bucket with water. When the bucket begins to overflow, stop the watch. If it takes two minutes to fill the bucket, that equals a flow rate of 2.5 gallons per minute. Fill the bucket in one minute—that is a flow rate of 5 gallons per minute. If the bucket fills up in thirty seconds, then the flow is 10 gallons per minute. Pretty easy. With humans, it's not so easy, it's more difficult and requires a bit more finesse. However, I did it, and so can you. Believe me, it is worth the effort to figure it out.

I started taking notice of my flow rate and decided to calculate it and then also turn the figures into some sort of chart so I can give myself a better understanding of what my doc was talking about, and here they are.

Before surgery output:	One year after surgery output:
No records before 20 seconds	14 seconds 12.5 oz or 367 Milliliters
	14 seconds 10 oz or 295 "
	18 seconds 15 oz or 444 "
20 seconds, 12 oz	20 seconds 17 oz or 500 "
22 seconds, 14 oz	22 seconds 18 oz or 533 "
25 seconds, 16 oz	24 seconds 20 oz or 590 "

Before surgery is approximately
18 MLPS

After surgery is approximately
24 MLPS

That's a 33 percent increase in the flow rate, which also lends itself to say I must have had at least a 33 percent loss in my flow rate over the years. Doctors actually have a system to measure urine flow rate. It's called uroflowmetry. In fact, you should really inquire about it.

There was an obvious and quite noticeable difference in exit flow rate after surgery. It was around two or three weeks after surgery when I went back into my doc's office to see Jeffery for another follow-up visit. He asked me about the flow difference I was experiencing now compared to before the surgery. I told him the difference. "It's like turning on the garden hose compared to before." He again leaned back and let out a loud laugh. I do wish I would have saved more data on the before-surgery flow rate; however, I probably just tossed it off to the side because those three listings above are the only ones I found amid my notes. However, in my defense, at the time I was recording all my data, I didn't know that I would be using it later in a book. I was more specific with the after-surgery data, as you can plainly see. Still, looking back at this information, it's quite evident that it took me a longer time to urinate less fluids. Something that I and most men do not even notice.

The human bladder, when in its normalcy, can easily hold sixteen ounces comfortably and tops out around twenty-four. The rate our bladders fill up depends obviously on the volume of fluids we take in. It has been several years since my surgery, and I can hold more now, but just after surgery and for several months, there was no way in the world I was ever going to hold sixteen ounces. In fact, six or seven ounces was at the high end of my threshold, and I made sure to make frequent trips to the restroom to ensure it never made it any higher. Obviously, it all depends on me keeping up with my Kegel exercises.

A very short Budd story: I did stress myself out, about a year and half year after surgery, one time while I was still doing all the recording of the time and ounces for the data above. I just wanted to see how good I was doing, and I made it all the way up to twenty ounces, but that was dangerously close to just exploding, and believe me, I was squeezing those sphincters to their max. I had to—I was driving in my car, and believe me, I was racing just to get home. I knew I had to record this one.

To be honest, the slowing down is so gradual, over so many years that I didn't detect a thing, and no man will until it's quite slow and obvious or it becomes painful—that's when we all begin to notice it. That's a hint for you; take notice now, and the easiest way to notice this slowdown is to monitor it. Also, just pay attention to others while you are in the men's room and doing your thing while they are doing there's. I'm not talking about looking at the guy next to you—that could get a little risky. I mean just notice the time for you and the guys all around you. My length of time standing at the urinal had gradually increased over the years. I just wasn't paying any attention to the time it was taking me. I just alerted you to this, so now you know and can't use my excuse. Because of my friends poking fun at me, I began to notice more than before that I would be standing at the urinal draining my antifreeze like I thought was normal, and the guy next to me would be done with his business and washing his hands, and I would just be finishing up. Although there is one good thing that comes with slow urination; I was the only one among all my buddies that could write his name in the snow. Once I started to take notice of the length of time, a small and scary item did come to my attention. I noticed at the end of my urination process, I would stand there even a little longer because I had to physically push out the last few squirts. It didn't just end like when I was younger; I physically had to push out the last squirts—not drips, but squirts. Which is another indication of the donut hole being squeezed down on the urethra. I'm not talking about the normal couple of pushes we all do after we are done. You know, the one extra push and perhaps that little shake at the end to get the hose fully drained. I'm saying about four extra pushes, and each one has about the same amount that came out. Here's how it went. After draining my fuel, I would relax and wait a second and then push out a squirt, relax, wait a second, and push, relax, wait a second, and push, and repeat this ordeal like four times. This is an obvious sign of the urethra closing down. When it begins to close down in size, not all the fluid will drain out of the bladder, which means a certain amount remains in the bladder—not healthy, said my doctor. It's bile fluid, and your body needs to rid itself of this material. Urinary tract infections may occur if our bladders are not drained correctly and completely, which is yet another telltale sign of the prostate. He told me to stand there as long as it takes and push out the remaining fluid, so that's exactly what I did, which means now, I was taking even a little longer while at the urinal. Tests, trials, and tribulations. Believe me, I was certainly going through them.

During this early part of my journey, the word "cancer" never came up in my doctor visits nor within our conversations, and to be quite honest with you, I never thought of that ugly word connected to me—not even once. At one of my regular six-month checkups, the doc explained to me that my prostate was still gradually getting larger, but slowly, plus my PSA results were still coming into him with slightly elevated results than the previous one, again a fraction of a difference. Well, more time passed, more doctor visits passed, and more PSA tests. Now, at this one particular point of my journey, my PSA results came back at 4.0, which is still in the normal range, but a small red flag did go up. During the next particular visit, my urologist expressed to me that he could feel my prostate gland was still continuing to get slightly harder than previous times, which meant it was not as soft as a normal and healthy prostate gland should be. While at this particular visit and still sitting on the table within his exam room, he showed me a few examples of what a normal and abnormal prostate gland looks like and what it should feel like. He explained to me the difference between the two sample glands. This visual aid really helped me to understand what my gland might look like at this point in my journey of time.

Many studies have shown that enlargement of our male prostate is clearly just a natural byproduct in men as we age, sort of like getting gray hair. Earlier, I discussed with you the donut shape of the gland. So now it makes sense; if you add the donut shape to the normal enlargement of the gland, it seems to be a standard MO that you would have a reduction in the urine flow rate. The most noticeable side effect you should be placing into your memory banks is there may be some trouble starting the stream of urine and even some dribbling or squirting at the end of urinating process, which I personally found out about as I stated a few paragraphs earlier. But wait, we aren't done yet; there is also the annoying few drips of urine that make it out much later into your underwear! Aging is such a fun experience. The reason the donut hole gets smaller is because all of the cells that make up the prostate get larger. As each one of the million tiny cells gets a little larger, naturally, the center hole will get a little smaller. The smaller the hole, the less volume and the less speed our urine will travel through the donut hole as it leaves us. It's all tied together.

It's time for some information you need to hear concerning the draining of a man's bladder. Because of the enlarging of our gland—no, wait minute. Now that you have been educated a little bit on the prostate gland and how it works, it's really not so much the enlarging of the gland that causes the problem. In reality, it's really the narrowing of the small hole within the middle of our gland that causes the associated problems. However, as the center hole shrinks in size, it naturally becomes ever more difficult for us to completely drain our bladder, which means there will be a small amount (small volume) of urine left stranded inside of our bladder. So after you are done draining your fuel tank and you think you have done your best, you will have to stand there for a few more precious seconds and try several more times to physically push out the remaining urine. If you don't take the time to stand at the toilet (or urinal) a little longer and do this extra trick—brother, bad news, this is what is going to take place. Because you left this small amount of liquid inside the bladder, your bladder fills up more quickly, making you feel like you have to urinate more frequently (just one more little sign of the prostate). One of the many docs I spoke with stated to me, when I use the restroom, to drain my antifreeze, I should take extra time and stand there after I think I'm done and relax for a moment and do about ten Kegel exercises to help better drain all of the urine (I'll explain more on Kegels later). Here's a good idea, and I'll pass it on to you. Right before I retire to bed for the night, I will use the restroom, drain my fuel, and then stand there for a few moments and try to relax my whole body. Once I feel relaxed, I will start to perform ten of my Kegel exercises.

This little trick flushes out most of the remaining urine that would normally be left inside the bladder. It would be good for you to also do this trick. Try to relax and do ten Kegel exercises whenever you use the restroom. Particularly at nighttime before retiring to bed, because if you make this a nightly habit, you might not have to make that extra middle-of-the-night restroom trip (yet another sign of the donut hole closing).

One more very important piece of Buddformation I will pass onto you, and I found this out quite by accident, but it works wonders and it came in quite helpful for me, so you can give this idea a try. I would reduce the amount of liquids I was taking in about two or three hours before going to bed, and sometimes, I would even totally stop consuming any type of liquids two hours before retiring for the night. This way, for the next couple of waking hours before going to bed, I was still draining the amount of liquid that my bladder was storing and not adding any more extra liquids to my bladder. It's the extra fluid you are consuming in the evening that will require the unwanted middle-of-the-night bathroom trip. So in conclusion, quit the intake and squeeze out the most you can.

Well, now back to the prostate. This involuntary enlargement of the prostate gland as we age is called benign prostatic hyperplasia (BPH). BPH is the most common prostate problem for men age fifty and up. Studies show about three million cases per year, also by the age of sixty, one out of every two men (50 percent) may be dealing with BPH. This next fact is ugly. By seventy-five years of age, nine out of ten men will have it! Again, it's not fun getting older? So here's another catch-22; even though BPH has several lousy side effects (urination difficulty which leads to infection, stones, or even reduced kidney function), again, BPH is not a sure sign of cancer, but you should know it might point to cancer. The good news here is BPH is not cancerous and BPH doesn't cause prostate cancer. The bad news is that BPH and cancer can happen at the same time. In all my research, I found no scientific studies, no hospital studies, and no doctors indicating a concrete reason for the cause of prostate cancer, which means no one knows how it gets into the gland in the first place. I'm not a highly educated professor, but when I look at the location of the prostate gland and see how far it is hidden deep inside of the body, that fact tells me it must not be coming from the outside world and most likely has to do with something inside the body.

My prostate, unknown to me, was gradually enlarging over the years, and it wasn't until I started a regular urologist six-month program that it was discovered. This discovery made it clear to me that millions of other men all over the world are probably in the same boat as I. Millions of prostates all over the world are gradually getting larger and harder over time, and we as men don't even know it. It's not publicized, it'd not advertised on TV, we don't even feel it and don't even have the slightest idea that it's happening. But the harsh reality is it is happening! When the symptoms or signs are noticeable and/or recognized, you must understand that you will already be many years into the enlarging process and didn't know it. However (and this is big), I continually went back to the same doctor for each of the prostate exams. The same doctor is important. This means my doc had my baseline, a starting point, so he knew me, he could feel that the gland was enlarging, and could feel the variations with each succeeding appointment. This is where you become important and the doctor becomes the common denominator in the equation; by visiting the same doctor/urologist over and over for your own prostate exams, your doc will be able to feel the same spot many times over the many years, so he can make his notes and will be armed with this knowledge. This is why he will be able to spot or, in better words "detect," all the subtle changes.

Take note of this: Even though enlargement and hardening of the prostate gland seems to be standard operating practice of our male bodies, both of these signs are still not positive signs of cancer. For it to be cancer, there are many other pieces of the puzzle that must come together before we start to have some anxiety. Some signs like the enlargement, the hardness, some difficulty in starting urination, slow flow rate, the all-important "PSA" reports, and your doctor's glove test are all pivotal pieces of information, and nowadays, there may be a few others medical pieces of the puzzle to add. However, and this is quite important, I did find out what the (MVP) most valuable piece of the puzzle, or in other words, the sharpest tool in the shed to use in helping detect cancer is, and that would be the prostate biopsy sample. This, my friend, is the real Sherlock Holmes detective in your journey. Some also called this method of diagnosing suspected prostate cancer as "the gold standard." We, as men, must pay attention to all the available signs, because all are important pieces of your health puzzle, a puzzle which you and your physician are slowly but accurately piecing together over time.

There is one piece of brilliant advice I came across, and I can't understand why this is not passed on to us guys as common advice, but unhappily, it is not. However, this book is about passing information onto you, and I must pass it to you right now, so listen up. My advice to you is to get all your PSA blood tests completed at the same lab each and every time, if possible. Here's the reason: Different labs use different testing methods and will use different machines in different locations and different lab technicians, all of which may result in different level readings coming back from these different labs and can lead to confusion for you and your doctor. Because of different labs, the doc may be getting conflicting results on all the paper work.

One more word of Budd advice: I don't know why this isn't also passed onto the patient before getting a PSA test done, because it wasn't to me, and it wasn't to a couple other gents either. However, I've read that ejaculation can artificially raise the PSA readings. This means if you have a PSA blood test schedule for you to preform, you should not ejaculate for two days before the test. Take that down in your notes.

Request an extra copy of all your PSA results for yourself and keep these extra copies in your own health records at your house. These reports are important for you to read, study, and understand, because you should be tracking your health history at the same time as your doctor tracks it. Listen, dude, it's your life, and they are your reports, so sit up and pay attention to them. If you are diligent in studying and tracking your own health statistics, you could possibly catch a red flag before your doctor does. I kept notes of whatever my doctor told me each time we had our regular six-month checkups. I also kept track of my PSA reports and watched as each one of them came to the doc with a very slight but higher level than the previous one. Get ready and believe me, brother, when I say this: Watching the levels creep up over time can be a great disappointment, but watch them, you must. If they come back with a no-change reading, it can be a wonderful thing; however, with my reports, not so much. My wife and I were disappointed when a 4.5 level report came back from the lab and so was my doc.

You know, I have read information in different books about different men sometimes having PSA readings of up to 15.0, and in rare occurrences, readings could reach as high as 50.0, but that high of a number seems to be quite infrequent! I've read and researched a lot of information about the prostate and spoken to men who were diagnosed with and braved through what I was about to go through. They made it, which gave me more confidence that I could make it too. I also listened to a couple of Sunday morning talk show programs on the radio devoted to this very subject. I learned, both the elevated PSA levels and the enlarged prostate together are still not a positive sign of cancer, which is good, but together, they really should raise both your doctors and your own concern about your health. This next statement is going to sound a little contradictory to what I preach in this book, but honesty is what this book is all about, and I feel I must report it to you. Some of the information I gathered during my research led me to believe that an enlarged prostate gland and higher PSA may not be as serious as some of the hype that's out there concerning the prostate (then again, there are always going to be the pros and cons to any subject matter). The side that I'm trying to show everyone is not so much the prostate pros-and-cons but, rather, the aftermath. Sure, I speak about the prostate and how it functions, what to look for, how to monitor it, and the signs to look at. But that's all information guys should know for good health. I'm stating the case that comes when you have a diagnosis of cancer, when the bony finger has already reached out and touched you. I want you to understand the seriousness of the situation you're in. It's not a game; there's no reset button. You don't get three chances and then you're out. I investigated many different sources of information concerning cancer, and with my family's background history concerning cancer, it all led me to believe it is a very serious situation, so when I found myself within that serious situation with my diagnosis, it scared the living daylights out of me.

OK, right about now, I'm thinking that many of you, as you are now reading about my journey, may be asking yourself this question. "Budd, if all your vital signs, like the doc's informational notes, the doctor visits, and glove test, and the slow urination and PSA reports, were pointing in this direction, and all the pieces of the puzzle were coming together, why in the world did you wait so long to get a biopsy?"

Well, I'll tell you why I waited. Part of the "why" is the bit of information in the above paragraph which states that this prostate stuff wasn't as serious as all the hype surrounding it. That small amount of info may have been a mistake for me to stumble upon because at first it played, all too well, into my procrastination nature. So adding that bit of info into the cast of characters for my procrastination show, you can see why I may have been dragging my feet a little and taking my time in the decision-making process during this whole thing. I was holding true to my continual postponement of things. I almost made a mistake because I was wrong to think such a thing. I was almost dead wrong. I should not have been avoiding the circumstances, I shouldn't have been procrastinating, and I probably shouldn't have been so confident in my laid-back thinking. You see, I thought what possibly a lot of men think: "Hey, I've been healthy all my life." "I'm young, strong and independent." "Why should I worry?" In retrospect, I wish I would have been a little more disturbed about all the pieces of the puzzle earlier on, because unknowingly, there was a dreadful monster who was silently going about his deadly craft inside me and wanting to take over my body for his own.

Also, in my defense, when one has been healthy all their life, as I was, and has a bit of a Neanderthal mentality, like I did, and all your vital signs are within the normal range and there's no large red flags or loud alarms that go off, there isn't any two-by-four piece of wood slapping you upside the head telling you to get your act together. Plus, when you start off in the totally normal range and all signs are A-OK, it may take many years to accumulate all the data from numerous doctor visits, glove exams, and PSA test results with all the information they contain because you only have an appointment at the doctors' office for a visit every six months—that's only twice a year. It does take time in order to see this puzzle coming into focus. None of the aforementioned items are overnight wonders with answers for a quick trip. Even though the PSA test results were coming back with a fraction of a point higher reading, that in itself wouldn't set off any alarms either. Remember, a 4.0 PSA test result is still considered to be within the normal range, and even a 5.0 is not a critically dangerous sign, and 5.0 still doesn't positively point toward cancer, but I feel it really should be a beginning point of getting serious with your doctor. Although I have read reports stating that some feel the real danger point starts at 6.0. Now, obviously the higher the level goes, the greater the chance of having prostate cancer. My own advice to all males, and I'm saying all this because I now have what is known as "hindsight," is to start acting when it reaches 4.0. A level of 10 or above is considered quite dangerous, and the presence of cancer can be great.

Plus, you should understand, in my beginning years, I wasn't doing any of my homework like reading up or studying about prostate cancer; I wasn't even thinking about it. Another reason, and probably the biggest reason it took so long, which I mentioned earlier, was the fact that I was once crowned the "king of procrastination" by some of my friends, and the old habit of dragging my feet showed itself once again. Another note in my defense is to remember that hindsight is always 20/20, so as you are sitting down and calmly reading all this book, it's like being a Monday morning armchair quarterback, which is OK. It's fine, because if the tables were reversed, I know that I would most likely be asking the very same question of you. It takes time to get all the ducks in a row, and at the time, I was just hoping and praying that, since everything was still within the normal range and there were no large red flags, everything would turn out to be OK. Everyone always hopes for the best, and I'm no different.

CHAPTER 2

My Biopsy

A nother six months have passed, and I am in his office for yet another visit. Again, this one turned out to be the same as all the previous visits, with the numbers up a fraction of a point over the previous numbers—not tremendously higher. Again, it was, just like before, a slow climb. After another six months slowly passed, and again, it came time for my golden glove test and to see the latest PSA test report. At this visit, the test report came back with a 5.0 reading, which meant this time it was indeed outside of the normal 4.0 range. Plus, it was the same for my prostate; it was a little larger/harder, so all signs were still moving in the same direction which they had been taking all along (the wrong direction). While all three of us were in his office (my doc, my wife, and myself), we began to look at each other. The look we all had was the look that we all knew. "It was time." My doc looked at us and made a statement that I didn't want to hear. This is what he said.

"We should now begin to think about taking a more strategic approach."

He explained that he would like to do a procedure called the transrectal ultrasound and biopsy of the prostate.

As I stated earlier, prostate biopsy samples are the real Sherlock Holmes detective in anyone's journey, and at this point of my journey, things were becoming a bit clearer. He explained the procedure could be done "in-house"—no hospital visit was necessary. The total time for this in-house procedure from when I walked into the office until the time I walked out would be just over an hour. I felt that nagging procrastination sneaking back into my mind as I sat there for a minute because, inside my mind, I was thinking, *Well, OK, but let's schedule the biopsy for some time next year*, but I knew right away I had to squash this thought for two reasons. One, my procrastination had to stop; and two, because my wife already had her calendar book out and was looking at different dates we had available, so I agreed and unenthusiastically said, "Let's do it." We all immediately agreed on two months instead of my year-out idea and scheduled the date. You know something, it kind of felt good to beat myself at my own game of procrastination.

All right, now for another little morsel of information which I learned the hard way and will pass on to you. Prior to a "transrectal ultrasound and biopsy of the prostate" (TRUS) procedure in your doctor's office, you will receive some detailed instructions concerning the entire procedure and, especially, the things you need to do before you go in. Please read the instructions completely, carefully, and most importantly, follow those instructions! I thought I read them completely and carefully, but I discovered later that I didn't follow them well enough. Around noon on the day "before" my ultrasound biopsy, I started getting a headache, which was slowly turning into an unpleasant migraine. I took two little, itsy-bitsy, tiny tablets to help ease my discomfort. Sounds OK so far. The next day, I'm in my doctor's office and ready to go through this procedure. While everyone there was getting prepped, including myself, I was being quizzed by the nurse. She has her little E-pad and checking off points as she was asking me a few of the normal questions like what vitamins, minerals supplements, or perhaps any medicines I had taken in the last forty-eight hours. Well, I didn't take any vitamins or mineral tables the day before, and I didn't even eat anything, which may explain my migraine. However, the nurse did ask me about medicines, so naturally, I mentioned to her about the two itsy-bitsy Advil Ibuprofen pills I took. *Wow*, talk about a crash and burn. I mean, it was like I pulled the electrical plug out of the wall socket of the television while everyone was watching the Super Bowl. There were moans and yelling (my wife does that when she upset). I felt so stupid at that moment. Those two tiny pills cancelled out the entire procedure, and I had to reschedule the whole thing for a later date. I wasted everyone's time—my doctor's time, the nurses' time, my wife took time off from her work for this procedure and, of course, my own time, all because I didn't entirely follow my well-structured and printed-out instruction sheet. Needless to say, nobody in the office, including my wife, was none too happy with me. I was totally embarrassed, just like a little puppy who gets in trouble and sticks his tail between his legs. I put my head down, put my tail between my legs, and left the office. My advice: Read and follow the instructions and just don't take anything like I did; it's not good. A few weeks passed, and once again, I was back in the doc's office for the ultrasound prostate biopsy. I was careful to reread the instructions and not take anything for forty-eight hours leading up to the procedure. I'm telling you, I ingested nothing but water this time. I certainly wasn't going to do that again.

I would like to take a moment here and describe to you just how the ultrasound and biopsy procedure played out for me, and hopefully, it will give you some insight of what to expect. Fortunately, it's not a difficult procedure. I was fully awake during the whole process. Of course, it starts off at the doctors' office, and once again, the nurse was asking me all those questions, only this time, it's before we go back, and also this time, I made sure there were no mistakes. This time, I passed the exam, and now, I was being led back to a small exam room to get prepped again. Things were going quickly, and before long, I found myself laying on an exam table on my left side, facing the wall, wearing nothing at all except my little white socks and a warm white sheet covering my body. I had not only reread the instructions but followed them completely, so this time, I was fully ready for the procedure. My doc came into the exam room and explained the procedure from start to finish. His good mannerisms made it sound simple enough. The doctor used a specially designed tool constructed just for this procedure. It has a handle at one end, which the doc holds onto and navigates along its merry route with a specially designed harvesting needle at the business end. In layman's terms, it is called a biopsy gun. When the doc pulls the trigger, it tells the super sophisticated snapping turtle needle, which is at the business end, to snip off a piece of prostate tissue and bring it back to the doc. Stop here for a second. The name "snapping turtle" is my own term for this. I don't know the precise medical name for it. Needless to say, but I'm going to say it, the snapping turtle needle is the star of the show. It does the job of removing all the tiny pieces of your prostate gland, which is then sent to the lab for biopsy examination, testing, and reporting. From these tiny pieces of our bodies' living tissue, which the lab truly scrutinizes, they can discover the presence of many diseases. Our prostate is pretty much centrally located within our pelvis region. It seems as if it is just as far in from the front as it is from our back side, and just as far up as it is down. Because of its centrally located position, the easiest way to reach our prostate and gather these biopsy samples is to follow a natural opening route. You are probably guessing the route right now. This is accomplished by inserting this tool (needle end first) into the rectum opening. So that is how it all begins. After inserting this device, the doc continues to move the snapping turtle tool upward and into the next larger rectum cavity and then navigates it to where it is extremely close to the prostate's location.

Once the business end of the tool is in this location, it is time for the tricky part; our prostate gland is located just beyond the outside of the rectal cavity wall, so once the needle is at this precise location, the doc will direct it to pierce through the anterior rectal wall membrane and find a spot on the gland that is favorable for a sample. At this point, the needle quickly snips off a very small piece of the gland and holds it within its jaws until the removal is completed. This snipping of the gland is repeated multiple times, obviously for multiple samples. I believe five samples were retrieved from my gland. Each sample, as it is extracted off our gland, will cause a small amount of pain, so be ready for this small pain. The doctors called this pain "mild discomfort." On a scale of 1 to 10, I would classify it right at a level 2 at the moment of removal. It is a little painful, but the pain and its discomfort are both very short-lived.

After one individual sample is extracted off the gland, it's pretty cool how the doc slowly navigates the needle to a new and different location and keeps extracting more samples. This specially designed needle is an incredibly cool piece of medical technology, but I feel compelled to tell you, even though it is a marvelous piece of technology, there is one drawback for the patient undergoing this procedure. When this special snapping turtle needle somewhat happily bites off a chunk of your gland, it makes a rather loud "click," and this clicking noise is both heard and felt with each tiny extraction. This loud clicking noise you hear is also quickly associated with the "mild discomfort" you may feel each time it merrily snips off another sample. It's sort of like listening to the musical theme from the movie *Jaws*. You hear the music and you know it is coming, but you don't know when. So here you are, laying patently on the table while the doc does his work, when suddenly, you hear this loud click and you feel the sudden pain, and then, as the pain subsides, you lay there, waiting in unwanted anticipation, knowing there's another *click* coming and also another bit of pain coming too, and just like in the *Jaws* movie, you hear the music but just don't know when it's going to happen; however, you know for sure that the shark is coming and someone is going to get bit. Once the doc feels he has enough extractions and the procedure is completed, your time is done, you can get dressed, and quickly head out of there, all the time hoping you don't have to go back into the oceans deep water anytime soon.

All those snipped off sample pieces are now swiftly sent to the pathology lab, where they are thoroughly examined inside and out. The pathologist, using their expert knowledge, will totally analyze and critically scrutinize each and every one of those samples. Here's something unfortunate; these pathologists are stereotyped as lab rats, but they are physicians the same as any other medical doctor (MD) and go through ten to twelve years of medical schools and residency. I think these guys get a bum rap being called lab rats; they are really great people, and I am sure they are the best at what they do. We should all be very thankful for them. They take great care in the importance of their analysis. Their findings are imperative to the decision-making process. This forensic lab researches all the individual samples for any type of disease that might be hiding within the samples. Here's something that you may not know, these guys also research for any "typical behavior" of any of the diagnosed diseases they may find. This "typical behavior" is important, because one needs to know how aggressive any disease might be. The more aggressive the disease, the more aggressive you need to be on your part to counteract it. I'll go a step further and say we need to be even more aggressive than that which is coming against us. Once the doc receives the pathology reports back in his office, he can successfully determine the next logical steps everyone needs to take. This process reminds me of a saying my father told me years ago which left an impression on me: "A wise man will study the ways of his enemy." I don't know where my dad got that saying, but when he told it to me, it really stuck. Believe me, those diseases are our enemy, and we need to study them well so we can unite together and fight a good fight so we can be bigger and stronger than that which is coming against us.

Well, let's get back to those samples taken from me. Great news! The pathology report for my sample biopsy came back clean. That's right, no sign of cancer! Can I get an amen, brother!!! Everyone was so happy, especially myself, that I decided to take my wife out for dinner to celebrate. I figured I could get back to my normal daily activities and shake off the fear which had been slowly building in the back of my mind. I never verbalized any of my fear, and neither did my wife, but I suspect she had some of her own. Both myself and my wife were very relieved to receive the all clear news. Nevertheless, still in the background and covered by shadows, there was something lurking inside of me, but for now, everyone was happy, and the sun was shining again.

Now, looking back on the whole situation, my doc wasn't so sure about the all clear news. I can see quite clearly now what my doc must have been thinking back then. He was thinking this. *Something just isn't adding up here.* Looking at all the signs, to him, things were a bit conflicting. He knew all my PSA results were coming back slightly higher each time I'm tested. He knew my urine flow rate wasn't quite right, it was a little slower than a normal person. In addition, the physical glove exam he was conducting on me twice a year did indicate a slightly larger and slightly harder prostate. Now, anyone of these items by themselves is not worrisome. Even so, when they are all bunched up together like mine was, it is something to be considered. My doctor was sharp; he knew all these signs which he was analyzing in his office were adding up and painted a picture, but they were contradicting the picture the pathology lab reports were painting. It's just that all things weren't lining up quite right. Again, I must thank God that my doc knew what he was doing and didn't just give into reading the pathology reports and making them his final word, which is just maybe what a procrastinator like myself would have been inclined to do.

Since all the samples of my ultrasound and biopsy lab reports came back clean and showing not to be cancerous, you can imagine how ecstatic I was. My wife and I were back in the saddle and riding into the sunset and going about our everyday lives with smiling faces. It's a great feeling knowing you dodged a bullet like this one. So for the most part, my life was good, and I actually stopped thinking about all the bad stuff that could have been. This beautiful euphoric feeling lasted only six months, because then, it was time for the next bi-yearly doctor visit. That's right, brother, even though the biopsy reports came back clean, it didn't mean the visits would come to an end and fade away. In fact, because it was such a close call, those twice-yearly visits became more essential, which is something else you should learn from my story!

CHAPTER 3

Diagnosis

At the end of those fun-loving six months, I found myself back at my doctor's office for the normal checkup and, I would like to add, with no worries, because remember, all reports came back giving me a clean bill of health. I'm having the normal exam with the normal questions and the all-important glove-test. Then I was off to my local LabCorp office for the PSA test, and of course, those results were sent to my doc. About two weeks later, his nurse called me and stated the doc wanted to see me. I was informed by my doc of my latest PSA information, and of course, it was again a fraction higher than before. That's when my doc said, "I'm sorry to put you through this, however, I think it would be prudent to acquire another physical biopsy ultrasound sample, only this time, I will strive to get them from an entirely different place and from a different location within the gland." By extracting different samples from different areas and further away from the previous location within my gland, it may produce different results. Well, I was set up for another rerun of the *Jaws* movie theme, and after this second ultrasound biopsy, there were only two things to do: pray a lot and try to wait patiently until the doc called me with the results. Well, big surprise, this time, the report came back, and bad news was awaiting me. The bold headline in the morning paper read: *Cancer Identified.*

This headline brings us back to the beginning of this book and the devastating phone call I received, which was the day Budd's earth stood still. The report was shocking, upsetting, disappointing. There are literally hundreds of ways to describe the feeling you experience when you hear those words for yourself and that cold boney finger is pointing directly at you.

I have always been a positive person (another trait from my dad), and I try to look at the brighter side of any situation. Now, understand I don't disregard or dismiss the bad. On the contrary, I totally try to understand it, but then, I also want to look up and try to understand where I'm at in the best light possible. I must tell you, this time, it was a very tough task for me to accomplish. However, the positive silver lining I did find within my bad situation was this: Because I had one clean prostate biopsy result (the first one) and one ugly result (my second one), there was this great possibility that the prostate cancer was small, and best of all, it was caught and identified at the earliest possible time it could have ever been caught. This ugly thing had been detected early which, again, I must reiterate, is the best possible time to discover it. The earlier it is caught, the more and various avenues of help there are, and this means the more tools you'll have to defend yourself with, which also means the better your odds are in totally defeating your enemy, and listen, my friend, that is a very positive silver lining to have in your favor.

When cancer's scrawny finger is pointing directly at you and your ears detect those heart-stopping words, within that one second of time, your life changes; from that moment forward, you are not the same anymore, your life is beginning to change and will continue to change. As I was listening to my doctor words during that historic phone call on that sunny day, as soon as those two words "prostate cancer" hit me, my eyes closed, a lump formed in my throat, and I didn't even hear the doctor's voice as he kept talking to me. His words coming out of the phone just slowly faded off into the distance as a thick emotionless fog of disbelief began to overtake me. I wanted to scream, but at that moment, my jaws seemed to be locked tightly together, but inside my mind, I was screaming, *No, no, no, no*. I remember that word echoing a hundred times inside my head. There also was this knot in my throat; I couldn't even swallow. I couldn't have spoken a word even if I wanted to. I'm not quite sure how long my mind checked out during that horrifying conversation; you don't have a sense of time during something like this because your mind is off the clock, but when my mind started to come back online, it was my body's turn to check out. I had no strength in my legs, and my knees weakened. My head felt so heavy, like it weighed a hundred pounds, as it fell forward and my chin hit my chest. I was still grasping the phone in one hand, as both arms fell to my sides. I had to sit down fast or I might just drop straight down to the floor. As I fell back into the chair, I just sat there, and this will sound strange, but my eyes weren't registering what they were looking at. It seemed as through my vision was inside my head as I was watching myself screaming, *No*, over and over. I could hear my heart beating inside my head and actually felt the pressure of the blood course through my body. The pressure started at the back of my neck, ran through my shoulders, and down my arms. It seemed to accumulate more pressure as it hit my fingers. The extra pressure in my fingers was probably due to the fact that I still had ahold of the phone and was squeezing it so hard. My body seemed to heat up, and when I finally began to regain some since of composure, I was able to raise the phone back up to my ear. Something else; at that moment, the phone sure felt heavy, I could feel the muscles in my arm as they forced the phone back up to my ear. I know all the words above were describing only about two minutes in real time, but to me during those moments, there wasn't any time; it seemed as if it was never ending. My doctor obviously had been through this type of phone call before. Bless his heart—he was waiting patiently for me to regain my composure. He knew what was going on at my end of the phone. He had just given the heart-wrenching diagnosis of cancer to another human being, and that can't be an easy task to live with. Heart breaking and world changing news to say the least.

The doctor explained to me what we needed to do next. His words were strong, calculated and straightforward. He said, "We both need to start making a few important decisions as soon as possible." When my dreadful phone call ended, my mind was still reeling in disbelief, the words *no, no, no* were still ringing inside my head. Thank God I was still sitting down because my body was physical trembling and I still felt very weak. Every part of my body—my arms, my legs—they all seemed to weight so much, they seemed so heavy. You know what's quite odd, you can't see words, you can't reach out and touch words, you can't feel them, but mere invisible words can take so much away from your thoughts and your life. I couldn't have gotten out of that chair and up to a standing position if I tried. Let me tell you something, at that moment, I felt like I was the only person on earth and nothing seemed to have any importance to me; time really did seem to stand still. Honestly, brother, nothing made any sense, and I was reeling in confusion and disbelief. My hands were trembling so uncontrollably I had to put the phone down or it was just going to shake out of my hand. During those few moments, I swear could have been looking out the window of my home and watching someone steal away with my car, and I honestly don't think I would have given it a second thought. You should know this fact about me; because of my family's past history with many cancers within different family members, over many years, inside my head, I honestly assumed the phone call I just received had given me a death sentence. At the time, I actually presumed I was reading the last chapter in the book, "The Life of Budd." Devastation mixed with despair would be mild words for what I was feeling.

At the time I received that devastating call from my doctor, I was obviously at home, but the positive part was, I was home alone. My wife was at work, and just speaking for myself, because everyone is so different in life and may handle situations differently, but being home alone was quite possibly the best way for me to receive this horrible news. For a lengthy period of time, I had a paralyzing feeling that only fear can bring on and felt sick to my stomach, a headache was developing, I didn't know what to do, didn't know what to think, my mind was all over the place, and even placing my hands into my pockets didn't stop them from trembling, I don't mind admitting this, but I was very afraid. It's a little difficult to describe in words how you feel at times like this, in particular to someone who has not gone through something similar. My vision was kind of in shades of gray—no real colors. Time seemed to be nonexistent. My mind was racing fast, literally bouncing from one thought to another and then to another, none seemed to have any meaning. Really, I didn't know what to do. It must have been about an hour later that I found myself pacing around inside my house with no direction or purpose; it was just the fact that everything was racing and my body had to move. I was in such a state of utter disbelief. In life-and-death situations, I've heard of people describe a feeling like they were standing outside their body, looking back at themselves, and it was similar to that feeling. I couldn't stop myself from trembling. Honestly, I thought I was going to throw up, and it was quite possibly two hours before my mind came back to making sense of my world.

Once my mind began to somewhat get back to thinking rationally, a few questions started to flood in like, oh my God, what do I do now? What's my next move? What shouldn't I do? Should I call my wife? Should I tell my family? Should I ask for their help? Could they possibly guide me through some of my next important life-changing decisions? A lot of big decisions would need to be made and carefully thought through. I also had thoughts like I should get my life's material items and paperwork in order so my wife would be OK if I wasn't here to help guide her through life. I really did have serious thoughts about me not being around to take care of her. I'm sure all these thoughts are quite normal to have during these times, and as each thought manifested itself, I would begin to think it through, but halfway into it, another new thought would take shape. It was one thought right after the other, and it was emotionally and mentally taxing. It was difficult trying to decide what actions to take, what direction to go, where, what, when, how… It is difficult to figure out the first step.

Perhaps you're now thinking about the first step you would take and, well, you should, because things happen unexpectedly in life. Another lesson I learned from my father was to look ahead and prepare for the unexpected, like saving for a rainy day or having enough food in the pantry for a couple of weeks in case a snowstorm hits. The first step for me was this. "I didn't do anything." Isn't it funny how my procrastination worked for my good in this situation? I didn't call my wife, I didn't talk to anyone; I kept it to myself. I replayed it over and over again in my head for hours. The tears flowed down my cheeks as my head and heart were filled with different emotions. I figure all the emotions I was experiencing were not unique to me but most likely were very typical for anyone in this spot. They are, of course, unique the first time it happens to you, but you know others have had the dreaded phone call and felt the same emotions. Well, the rest of that day, my mind just reeled back and forth from one extreme to the other. Some maddening thoughts are just mindblowers. It's so bizarre how your own mind and the thoughts within us can make your pulse rate climb and your heart rate quicken and give you a headache all at the same time. The entire day seemed to be one long, drawn-out bad dream. I just wanted to wake up in a different day, in a different time, on a different planet.

Of course, this elongated day did pass, and yet another difficulty presented itself to me. As I was pacing around the inside of my house, I glanced at the clock, and my wife was due home within the hour. I knew right away that I wasn't going to tell her anything about the phone call I received. I couldn't bring myself to tell her or anyone else, for that matter. I wasn't yet able to handle it myself, so how could I break this sort of news to her? I knew I had to get a handle on it before breaking the news to her or anyone. I'm her rock, I'm her shield; I can't show her my fear, my confusion. If I did, I would fall apart again, so until I had a grip on the situation at hand, this news stays put. For the present, I would keep this horrific news to myself and deal with it for a short while. I needed to wrap my own mind around what was happening to me and deal with the situation before I proceeded to tell anyone. The real test for me at this present time was to come to my senses and put on a happy face before my wife's arrival. Because when she walked through that door, I needed to appear to her as normal as I could, I needed to look at her, to talk to her, hold her hand, do everything I normally do, to make her feel that all was good in "Budd Town, USA." I washed my face, shaved, combed my hair, and even put on a clean shirt. I did the best interpretation of my happy self, while inside, I was not even close to being myself, and I still felt sick to my stomach. Fortunately for me, the timing was good. I greeted her at the door and even our dinner went smoothly. My wife was tired after a stressful day at work and wanted to curl up with the book she had been reading and just veg-out at home while leaving the hectic work-a-day world behind her. This was wonderful news for me! It allowed my heart to slow down and keep my thoughts to myself. I realized today I would not have to look into those beautiful eyes of hers and tell her any bad news; I could spare her feelings for another day. Those eyes, by the way, are almost always able to see right through my shenanigans. She read her book for a while. Later, we got ready for bed, and quite fortunately for me, the evening took care of itself.

I ended up taking a sleeping pill to help me sleep. I knew my racing mind and sprinting heart would not allow me any sleep tonight. When the morning alarm woke us, I knew what I had to do. I got dressed quickly and acted natural, trying my best to not let my voice crack. I acted like I was eating while we were having our breakfast cereal, made some small talk, and occasionally placed my hands under the table because my fingers were again beginning to tremble, my stomach was in knots, and I wasn't even the least bit hungry. I had to fake it and put on a cheerful face so my wife wouldn't think anything was amiss. I warmed up her car before she left for work and watched as she drove away. I just wanted to be alone with my thoughts and also be secure inside my home and figure out this problem. I needed more time to think and figure a few things out. As she left for work that morning, I watched her car fade into the distance, and once I knew I was truly alone, I walked back into the house. When I turned to close and lock the door behind me, it all seemed a bit weird, like I was in a slow-motion movie, you know, like when you are doing something but your mind is in some other state. After closing the door, I still remember that solitary yet seemingly loud *clank* as the deadbolt snapped into the locked position. That *clank* seemed to echo a dozen times throughout my head. I stood at the door, like my shoes were glued to the floor, and stared at my hands, one on the doorknob and one still holding tightly onto the deadbolt handle. I didn't move a muscle; my mind was again racing, I knew my blood pressure was building because I could feel it, but my body seemed frozen. I was now alone and didn't really have any idea of what to do or how to get started. I don't know how long I stood at that door still holding the handle, but it wasn't until a few tears fell onto my forearm that I gradually came back to reality.

I'm now home alone, and I began to feel the weight of the problem start to press down on me. It may sound like a cliché, but it really did feel like a huge physical weight was on my shoulders. I just sort of aimlessly wandered through the house. That early morning was a fog, and just like the day before, time seemed to stand still and the hours just stretched on at a slow pace. I ended up in our bedroom as my problem seemed be growing heavier. I can't tell you if I had anything to eat, because at times like this, some things just don't have any importance. I do remember, while pacing around the bedroom, that the feeling of being lightheaded began and the strength began to leave my knees. I had to sit down. We have a cushiony chair in our bedroom, so I dropped into it. My vision began to cloud from the buildup of tears, and that's when the enormity of the situation settled in and I started to cry.

I'm rather a normal guy, height 5'11 and 165 lbs., and like most guys, I think of myself as just on the "macho" side of life. Friendly and outgoing, I have always enjoyed the outdoors, expressly enjoy walking in the rain and getting soaked to the skin by a million raindrops. Funny how tiny each one of those little raindrops are, yet when enough of them fall, you get soaked down to your underwear, that is, if you're wearing any. I enjoy working in the yard, doing a few sports, driving 4x4s, camping in the woods and, of course, cars. Yet that morning, in that chair, while I was crying, I must have looked like a little boy who just lost his lifelong friend—his dog. I wasn't only crying, man, I was wailing. The tears would not stop! Because of my family's past history of multiply cancer deaths, I really thought the phone call I received was the end of me. I must have sat in that chair for hours, weeping and worrying. I prayed for help and guidance from the big man above and kept playing different scenarios over and over again in my head. I mean, how does one begin to tell his wife this kind of news? How can you prepare your mate for something like this? What do you say and where do you begin? While curled up that morning in my bedroom chair, I must have cried myself to sleep, because the next thing I knew, I was waking up to the ringing of the phone and a cramp in one leg. My heart actually jumped, because at first, I thought it might be my doctor calling again. I simply wasn't ready to receive another medical news flash inside a horrible phone call. Thankfully, our caller ID showed that it was my wife's office, so I took two deep breaths just to help compose myself before picking up the phone. She was calling to say hi to me during her lunch and to see how my day was going. I must tell you here that my wife is a sweetheart of a woman. I did good on the phone. I kept the news in and made sure my voice didn't betray my dreadful secret. We exchanged some pleasantries, and she was happy. I had to keep it short because I was almost breathless by the time the phone call ended.

The afternoon rolled on, and honestly, it was pretty much a haze too, although I did have moments during the day to organize a few of my thoughts and also begin to think about a plan. Once again, as I looked at the clock, it was getting closer to the time for my wife to be leaving her work. I started to compose myself again. You guys know the drill: wash up, comb hair, put on a clean shirt. I had to make it look like it was a "good day in Budd Town," hoping it was going to be a smooth evening. She called and said she would be a little late—all the better for me. Dinner went well, dishes got washed, and the rest of the evening went as planned. I acted like nothing was wrong. Nobody was the wiser, although inside, I was panicking and screaming, although the difference for today was I had some time to walk through my situation, a little time to think about it, to plan, my problem was getting a little easier to deal with.

The next morning, I again watched my wife drive off, walked into the house, closed the door, turned the deadbolt handle, and heard that loud click. As I felt the weight again start to come upon me, I squared my shoulders and said, "No," to myself. I didn't want to feel defeated anymore, I didn't want this weight on my shoulders, I didn't want to walk around in confusion and disbelief again.

Honestly, it felt like my dad was standing right there next to me, placing his hand on the back of my neck, telling me, "Straighten up your shoulders, son. This is where you need to start figuring out how to deal with the problem that has come against you." My dad had many quotes. I wrote most of them down so I could save them. I call them "Odin-isms." One special quote of Odin's was, "it's not the problems that attack you in life but, rather, how you counterattack those problems that will define you as a man." My dad's wisdom was always simple and, quite honestly, straightforward yet profound. Thanks, Dad, for helping me get started on this problem, and now, I had to face it head on. At this point, and with this problem, I knew what I had to do. I had to figure out when, where, and how to tell my wife. She's my partner in life, and she deserves to know. She will have to live with any of the consequences no matter the outcome. My wife, my partner, my life—we are extremely tight. We know each other well; we talk with each other and share everything. I was actually surprised that I was able to keep this from her like I did; she's good at seeing through my escapades. I also had to think about the best way to tell my family. I had to begin looking forward, head up, not down, and taking the next important steps in this journey.

At times like this, you can fall down and cry if you like or if you need to. It's OK, there nothing wrong about doing that sort of thing. I did it, but then, after a while, stand up tall and look the problem in the eye and say, "You aren't going to win today." If you have been confronted with a cancer diagnosis, you might take my advice and think things over for a while and formulate a plan for yourself before throwing it out into the universe for all to see. I think those first few days which I spent keeping this misfortune to myself and thinking things through in my own mind at a very raw level really helped me to deal with the situation and, quite possibly, helped me confront it head on. Nevertheless, I've dealt with this life-shocking news alone and for long enough; it was time to open up and talk to my wife, explain it to my family, and seek my doctor's professional advice. After all, they're all here for me, they will want to help and, quite possibly, may be my greatest associates throughout this battle for my life. That's exactly what it is too—a battle, and it's for your life.

All right, it's once again late in the afternoon. It's about an hour before my wife is due home from work. I've thought about my situation with a clear head, and I also have come up with a rock-solid strategy of how to inform my wife. It's all planned in my head, just how to tell her and at the precise time, so it should go smoothly. I have played this plan over and over on that big movie screen inside my mind. First, I'm going to clean up real nice. Second, I'll have a nice dinner all prepared and ready to eat when she walks through the door. With a nice tablecloth and a couple of candles to make it romantic and soothing, we'll take our time during dinner, and I'll tell her how much she means to me. Third, after dinner, I'll give her some time alone to do all the little things she always does at home around the house after dinner. While she's doing her assortment of evening things, I'll start my deep breathing exercises so I can get through my speech without choking up. When she's ready, both of us will sit down on the couch to relax a bit and converse about our day. I'll take her hand in mine and calmly begin to explain the whole situation, starting with the doctor's phone call. This was a brilliant plan, and I really thought it would go off without a hitch. Well, I must tell you, the first part of the plan worked great, and then it of course fizzled quickly. I was all cleaned up, and we did have a nice romantic dinner, and I even began my breathing exercises. However, this is where my plan totally fell apart. My plan crashed and entirely burned to a crisp. My wife threw a monkey wrench into my main gears, and the whole thing went up in smoke.

This is what happened. I was ready to move to the couch, sit down with her, and deliver my well-thought-out speech. No such luck. As she finished up her things, she turned to me and causally said, "You know, honey, I really thought we would have heard from Doctor Cowan's office by now." As soon as those words were off her lips, and almost before they hit my ears, she stopped cold in her tracks, man. I mean, like she just froze, and I knew my well-laid plan just hit a big snag. She turned toward me, stared right at my eyes (like an eagle looking at its prey), and asked in a very rigid tone, "Did he call you?"

Bam! That question and the way she clearly laser focused it at me confirmed the fact that she knew me pretty well. At that moment, my failsafe plan ended. I mean, the Hindenburg lasted longer. My heart was already beating faster than normal, and my mouth wouldn't work. I tried to swallow so I could say something, but that didn't work either, because halfway down, my saliva turned into a rock and locked up in the middle of my throat, and I could hardly breathe. My vision of her was beginning to get blurred because the tears were already filling my eyes, and at that very moment, my wife knew I had cancer. We both just stared into each other's eyes and didn't move. Time wasn't just slowing down; it once again stopped. We locked ourselves in a tight embrace, and we both cried. Neither one of us said a word for the longest time. I was trembling so much that she could feel it, so she held me even tighter.

After a few moments, we looked at each other, the emotions started all over, and more tears flowed. I really don't know how long it was 'til I was finally able to take a deep enough breath to begin to speak, although my words were crackly. We held hands, and I slowly began to tell her about the terrifying phone call, and believe me, it was difficult to get the words out and still breathe at the same time. It was an extremely life-challenging moment, only this time, it was for both of us.

I held this in for a few days and was able to grab ahold of my ordeal, and now it was time to have someone next to me who wanted to help shoulder this challenging problem that life threw at us both and weighed so heavily on me. Now, this may sound a little selfish of me, but after I told her the whole story, it felt really nice to be able to talk about it and feel someone else help me shoulder some of the weight. Valerie was not only glad to be here with me and for me, but she wanted to help and do anything and everything she could. She is an immensely wonderful soulmate. I can honestly say that I will love her forever no matter what the future holds. Something else to interject here—I have no idea how a goofy guy like me ended up with such a wonderful, caring, intelligent, and sweet person as Valerie. It's one of life's little mysteries.

My advice to other guys facing this same situation: First, think it over for a short time, because it's something you need to confront and wrap your mind around. You may need a little time for the severity of the situation to be processed. Second, get a close supporter, whether it's your life partner, a super friend, or family; get someone who is near to you and that you can trust. You are now faced with some huge, difficult, life-changing decisions. These three words, "life-changing decisions," used to mean something a bit different to me e.g. getting married, buying a house, or starting a family. Well, brother, my reality and my perception changed with just one phone call, in just one afternoon, from just one doctor. Now, don't get me wrong here, getting married, buying a house, and starting a family are still life-changing decisions, but they're more like walk-in-the-park decision compared to the decisions someone is faced with when the word "cancer" punches you in the face. Find someone to help with these substantial life-transforming decisions. It's naturally going to be overwhelming because of the uncharted territory you'll find yourself in. There will be a multitude of choices to explore and different paths you can take, and you must deal with them all. You must look at each one carefully. It takes time to go through this process, and at times, it will be exhausting. You will be dealing with your health, your life, and your future, and at these times, you'll find that your own mind may be reeling from the overwhelming information and decisions you're faced with, which means you may not have all your own brain-power at your disposal. A second brain is very helpful; somebody who is loyal to you and may help in selecting the right path to travel. A helpmate is extremely valuable. There is help on the outside as well—others who have dealt with this matter and people like doctors or books, guides, and different medicine. Remember, you do not have to go through this alone. There are external resources for you. You might find these following few words as help too: "In a multi-tude of counselors, you shall find wisdom." I was fortunate, for I had three close people, and clearly, the primary one is and will always be my wife, Valerie. I truly believe she would give her life to save mine. The day Valerie came into my life, heaven gave up an angel and I acquired one.

Another qualified confidant of mine who was quite unexpected but very much appreciated, and he's a good friend of mine, Mr. Frank Lopez; he was a great influence. When my buddy Frank heard about my situation, he was incredible. He got right up in my face and said, "Why aren't you at the doctor right now? You call your doctor, you call the hospital, call anyone and everyone you need. I'll even help, but get in right now and get that cancer out of your body and do it as soon as possible."

Obviously, Frankie provided me with a little different viewpoint on my situation. He gave me something I didn't have before. That something was exactly what my procrastination kept hidden from me: a sense of urgency, a good kick in the pants, so to speak, kind of like my dad would have done too. Because of my procrastination and somewhat clouded mind at the time, I didn't see it before. I can say that Frankie gave me a good kick-start. You see, Frank has personally experienced the effects of cancer in his family and was fully aware of the severity of it. So let me pause here for a moment and say, "God bless you, Frankie, and thank you again."

My third helper was Charlotte, my sister, who personally knew friends who went through this and provided guidance.

Besides those three main helpers I mentioned, there were many others who also came to my aid, and each one of them gave me an extra boost of "go-juice" for my journey. I have tried to personally thank everyone for their assistance, but if I missed you and you're reading this, I want to thank you right here. It's truly amazing how much support a person receives when they are confronted with life-changing adversity and needs help from others. It's rewarding and also quite humbling.

Cancer, it's one of those horrifyingly ugly words that carries with it a life-altering understanding. Honestly, I'm not the same person that I was before the day I received that paralyzing phone call and heard those life-shaking words and most likely never will be the same person ever again. I went through a life-threatening journey. Cancer was on its way to claim another life; however, prayers and technology won out. Like other cancer survivors, they will all surely understand when I say there's a place inside your mind that brands you and makes you look back at the past because you have been touched with such misfortune and adversity which cancer can surely put a person through. It also makes you turn to the future with brighter anticipation but looking at the positive side, and the best of all, the experience gives you an excellent appreciation of the here-and-now side of life. Sure, I can laugh at the same things as before and I look the same, but inside my mind, there is a shadow in the background lurking around, and I'll never forget it. I'm one of the lucky ones to be known as a survivor. Uncertainty and hesitation are present because I understand that life can take an unexpected turn, but I want to see the good in life and understand all the beauty there is while I'm here. I don't feel like I'm the same happy-go-lucky, who-cares-what-happens-next type of fellow that I was before the phone call. Life now has a more serious side for me. When I say a "more serious" side of me, please understand I'm not saying I'm the old man in the corner that never smiles—just the opposite. I want to be more serious about appreciating the world around me and the beauty it beholds. I can honestly say that I just "want to celebrate another day of livin.'" I feel a need to enjoy life more than I used to, and all moments are more valuable to me as I am sure they will be for you. Simple things, like the enjoyment I find in surveying my beautiful, green, freshly mowed lawn (love that fresh green smell). Or when I watch my lawn sprinklers spreading their sparkling drops of moisture in the morning sunshine because they look like small liquid-glistening diamonds of nourishment for the grass. My journey reminded me to look at the value of living in the moment, because it finally clicked in my head—the moment is all we really have. A month ago, a day ago, or even a second ago is gone. It's in the past, and there is no way to change it, and we all know the future is out there, but the future never really comes, because when it gets here, it's no longer the future, it's now the moment. It's similar as looking at the dates on a tombstone. You have the date the person was born and you have the date they passed away, but if you look at the dash between the two dates, you can see a life time of moments. When the sky is a beautiful shade of blue on a warm sunny afternoon and I find myself in the backyard, sipping a cold glass of freshly brewed iced tea, I think, *Ah, life is good*. The littlest things sometimes scream out to me, "Life is a serious moment. Live it now and enjoy it now." You never really know when or how fast it might change. This life-changing journey left me with a new value for life, and when that value hit me, it hit hard, and trust me it left a large impact crater. Here's an example of how I look at life a little differently. Today, when I find a small bug inside my house (my environment, where I belong), instead of seeing that bug as an enemy and killing the little guy with bug spray or my shoe, I find myself capturing it in a small box or tissue paper and taking it outside to release it into the grass (its environment, where he belongs). When I release that little bug so he can live another day in his environment, I'll look up toward the sky and say to the big guy, "Thanks for doing that for me." Live your purpose. Help others live theirs...

I can tell you this: if you have been diagnosed with any type of cancer, do not ignore it, don't turn your back, find out all you can about the category, the type, the size, everything you can; it will become a matter of life and death. Begin to fight it immediately!! This internal and silent monster does not get smaller, it doesn't take a day off, and it certainly does not fade away. The cancer has a journey also, and its goal within its journey is to grow silently inside of you (silently, because it doesn't want you to know it's there). It wants to take over what it does not own, it wants to steal your life away, and unfortunately, and I have to say, it seems to be good at it. The cancer can get bigger, stronger and, worse yet, become more aggressive.

Here's an uninteresting and ugly fact. At the time of my surgery, prostate cancer was the second leading cause of cancer death in American men. I'm not sure, but it may have moved to third place recently. If the cancer is large enough to be detected, then it is also large enough to be of real danger to you, which means your future may be in real peril. Just ask my friend Paul. Wait a second, we can't ask him. Please understand that I'm not trying to scare anyone here, but I am trying to alert you to give you the proverbial kick in the pants. I'm trying to give you real-life experiences I had and real facts that I have learned, facts that need to be addressed, not passed over or ignored like I was willing to do at first. I wanted to ignore the situation as if, somehow, it would just fade away. I didn't want to look it straight in the eye like my father would have. Another lesson I should have learned earlier from Odin Thor is to stand against that what comes against you.

Although my doc (Cowan) did not openly mention the word "cancer" during any of my early initial doctor visits, I bet it was in the back of his mind. He is very knowledgeable and has been trained to detect it. His years of experience are noteworthy. The most likely scenario is he might have been trying to spare me from becoming fearful before we had all the facts, which I can appreciate. Most of the information I've gathered from the many books, pamphlets, brochures, and other resources which I researched did mention prostate cancer, which is good because you need to be thinking in the right direction and have all possibilities laid out for you to help and assist in making the wisest decision for the situation you may find yourself in. Earlier, I mentioned the radio talk shows that I listened to, and one fact that was included into both talk shows was this statement. The doctors stated that more men die with some amount of prostate cancer present in their bodies than men who actually die from prostate cancer. Hold on, we need to stop right here, right now. *Do not* take that one statement and run with it as an excuse to delay any further doctors' visits, testing, or investigation. If you have positively been diagnosed with prostate cancer, it's my personal recommendation, that you eradicate it ASAP. Take whatever steps necessary and do it with the utmost urgency. The sooner the better, because cancer will not go away on its own accord; you have to fight it. That's right, the cancer and you are in a fight—a battle for your body. The cancer has but one goal, and that is to be the champion. It grows faster, bigger, stronger, and begins to take over your body and then your life. So, brother, eradicate it ASAP because you don't want the cancer to be the champion. Here's a hint: If the cancer becomes the champion, what do you become? The loser. Don't let that happen.

Here's a surprising fact you might want to consider and make a note of. There are *no early warning signs*. Yes, there are signs, and we all call them early warning signs, but in reality, when we begin to detect what we ourselves and the medical culture call "early signs," they are early for us, but they are not early for the cancer. When cancer is detected, believe me, this assassin has already been there for a while, you just didn't know it. What we call early signs only show that the cancer has already got his shop up and running and even hung a few "open for business" signs in the window, which means he been there for a while, and those are the signs we see, and we all call them early signs. Sadly to say, sometimes they are too-late signs.

You can be sailing merrily down the river of life, feeling great and feeling healthy while this silent assassin is beginning a deadly assault on you. That's exactly how I was sailing, on calm seas and feeling good too. Prostate cancer, as well as any cancer, has a "run silent, run deep" method of operation. I would categorize it as stealthy, because it can run under the radar for a while. Like I mentioned, it can grow slowly and silently. You don't feel any pain when it starts up, and you don't feel it growing inside of you. In the very beginning, there are no lumps, bumps, bruises, pain, or red flags to see or to feel, which would tell you absolutely something is amiss. It hides from sight, hides inside your body, and just hangs out. It will slowly grow in size until it can reach out and grab the outside wall of the prostate. Once it breaches the outside wall and escapes into the bloodstream, it uses our human body bloodstream to travel around like a free pass on a long slow train ride. Once this enemy is outside the gland, this thing can run ragged and perhaps find another spot to set up another shop for business with a sign in the window, and perhaps this next spot or area of the body may not be as easily detected. I'm certainly not meaning to alarm anyone reading this, I just want to share with you some facts and opinions of how serious the situation can become if untreated. I read in one piece of information that one of the off-spring of prostate cancer may just point to bone cancer—not good, my friend. Any form of cancer also may spread to nearby lymph nodes or the liver. Get familiar with the medical terms associated with any cancer so you can speak with the doctors using their own vernacular to communicate with them intelligently. They will appreciate it.

If you have been diagnosed with prostate cancer or, for that matter, any type of cancer, below are the following questions I found out about and you might want to ask too:

How much cancer was found? Doctors might call it the "volume" of cancer. More volume usually means a more aggressive cancer. Low volume a bit more time to scrutinize the treatment options. High volume=less time; you must deal with it quickly. We found the cancer as soon as it really could be detected, my recorded volume was low. Volume means the percentage of the prostate taken up by the cancer.

Ask about the Gleason score of the cancer? When I went through my journey, there was low, intermediate, and high. The fact that I was diagnosed early within my journey also lead to a classification of a Gleason score 6—a low grade and less aggressive. A Gleason score of 10 is high grade. However, one book of information stated that the traditional Gleason scoring of cancer is going to be phased out over several years. Just check with your doctor.

Would a bone scan or CT scan or even a PET scan be beneficial to have completed? Some different types of scans may be able to detect whether the prostate cancer has spread. If the PSA is higher than 11, a bone scan might be performed. A bone scan does not really show the cancer itself (I wish they did); instead, they can show the area of bone growth associated with the cancer. Bone scans to me seem to be right out of a Star Trek movie because of the technology which is used. A miniscule amount of a nuclear substance is injected into the body and races through the bloodstream. Our human bones absorb this substance. Once it is absorbed inside the human bone material, the scanning mechanism can detect where it is inside the body which, in turn, shows up on the final picture. These bone scans will help by showing the doctor any "hot spots" that may suggest the cancer has spread to the bones. This may be the worse-case scenario in spotting cancer, but it's worth asking about. Years ago, doctors used x-rays to help detect cancer; however, this radioactive scan technique detects cancer earlier and more precisely. Modern technology is so cool.

What stage is the cancer? Cancers are graded using different scales however one of the many scales used is known as stage. I believe that there are typically five stages to this cancer, and the doctors like to know what stage it's in to best define the treatments. Stage 0, 1, 2, 3, and stage 4. Any and all information you learn about this cancer can be useful in fighting this deceitful enemy, and fight you must, because it's fighting against you every minute of the 24-hour day, 7 days a week, 365 days a year. It doesn't rest or take coffee breaks.

What is the time or "window of opportunity?" What is my particular situation before the cancer might spread outside the prostate? This might be particularly helpful if you have a cancer grading which comes back as high grade, because high grade means you move fast. OK, guys, let's just stop for a moment right here. Listen up and be smart; this window question is actually a problematic question and a very speculative question to answer, and most doctors will not answer it because there's a lot of uncertainty built within the question itself. But ask it anyway and then back it up with a side question like, "I know this question is difficult to answer, but perhaps you could give me your professional and educated guess of time based on the evidence we have in front of us and from the biopsy reports, your past experience, and also your expert knowledge on the subject." Like three months, six months, a year. The diagnosis date is obviously the date the cancer is detected, or in other words, your start date, and when it breaches the wall to exit and find another spot, that would be the end date. Well, the time between the two dates would be the "window." See if the doc has some idea based on the lab results about volume and grade. Even a guess about the window of opportunity is better than nothing at all. A guesstimate concerning when the cancer is more likely to spread is just an educated guess, but it's better than none. Be smart enough to know there isn't a doctor in the world that would ever say something like the following: "Since the cancer was discovered on March 10, seven months from now, on October 10, the cancer will make its move, so our window of opportunity is seven months." You may get a pathology lab test response indicating that the volume is low so you have more time, maybe years. There is no precise timeline, but an estimated guess helps.

Doctor, is there perhaps a chance, just a chance, that someone else's biopsy test results might have gotten mixed up with mine? This question is a long shot, and to be totally honest, this rarely happens, but truly speaking, this is not unheard of. If anyone has any reservations at all, a second biopsy is a good idea, even though it means another *Jaws* movie to sit through.

Doctor, do you think it would be prudent to get another biopsy from different locations within the gland? Was the cancer found in just one area or multiple areas?

Grab a pen and write this next question down, it's my last question for you to ask, it's an important and excellent question too, because you need to know the answer:

Doctor answer me this. If perhaps I choose a particular procedure and that procedure doesn't work and the cancer does reappear, what then? The procedure doesn't matter at first, because you need to ask this question with any and all procedures that you have to choose from. The answer you receive should influence you greatly to choose (or not choose) a particular procedure. No matter which way you decide to rid yourself of this monster, there will be an aftermath, so once the procedure is completed and you are traveling down life's road once again, you need to be aware of what may happen later on, like perhaps a year from now or two years from now. This happened to a dear friend of someone I know. Two years later, it came back, and he could not redo his treatment. Unfortunately it is a reality of life. When you ask this question, what you are really looking for and what you are trying to find out is to make sure there is no dead-end streets on the path you take. I found out if the route you choose doesn't work totally and this ugly menace comes back, sometimes, you are out of options. Some procedures provide for an alternate route or, in other words, "a second chance," and unfortunately, some procedures will *not* allow you to try a second time or even a second avenue. You have to understand that, sometimes, if you pick one route and it doesn't work, you can't go back later and pick another one; they don't all work that way. You want to investigate and find out what all your options are in case it happens to you later. Down the road, if the procedure you are leaning toward fails and the monster returns, you don't want to learn the answer to this question after it is too late.

Find out before and this answer should affect your next move. This is a good lesson I learned from my dad. He would tell me, "Never box yourself into a corner, son. Always look for an alternative route or a second chance—an alternate way out." You not only need to research very diligently all the procedures that are available for you to defeat this deadly menace but also what the second chance is in case your first choice fails, and, brother, some of them can fail. An important question, it could pay big dividends later. Write that one down!

On a lighter note, here's a lesson I learned from my pastor: Under no circumstances do you ever want to call this ugly menace "my cancer." Like saying my house, my car, my shoes, calling it my cancer, means you own it. You do not own this ugly and dark thing, brother; this is not something you want, so don't claim it. Refer to it as "the cancer." It's not yours, and believe me, you don't want anything to do with it. This thing is your enemy, and its goal is to somehow end your life. The reason I'm telling you not to call it "my cancer" is simple, this battle that you now find yourself in is not only a physical battle against cancer for your body, it's also a mental battle, and you should remain strong on both fronts. Choose your words carefully, brother. Words are powerful. Fight the good fight of faith. OK, I just gave you a few questions to ask your doctor, and hopefully, you may have a few questions of your own which I didn't list above, but go ahead and ask your doctor anything you want to. Ask as many questions as you like—it's your body, it's your life, and it's your fight. Remember this: There are no bad questions. It's your body, and you need to know all the information available concerning this battle—the good, the bad, and the ugly. Brother, it's a tough journey, and you need to be ready, which also means you need to know the best information and the best technics available to you, and you should unfortunately know the worst-case scenario too so you can do battle the best way possible. You were just dealt a bad hand in the card game of life with this diagnosis, so no question is stupid. Face it and defeat it. Listen to everything with an open mind to make the best educated and calculated decision possible. Your doctor will appreciate your openness and honesty, and you should make many inquiries if he doesn't like your questions or all the inquiries. My advice to you: Get a different doctor. There's a ton of them out there to choose from.

Space for your notes:

CHAPTER 4

Treatment Options

Now we'll be moving a little further along in my journey, and we will discuss a few treatment options I was faced with. Even though the primary step of any journey is usually the first step which gets the ball rolling, but it's usually the smallest step to take when compared to the other steps you must complete; however, the proverbial first step is always considered the most important step of all. It's the needed step that gets the gears turning. Like turning the key or pushing the button to start your car, turning the key or pushing that start button in itself is just a minor step, but you have to admit it's the primary step for the journey. Once the car is started and the engine is hot, you can begin revving up the *R*'s and dumping the clutch. From that moment on, you have to hold on tight and go for the ride. Compare it to turning on your computer. Turning it on is a minor, almost trivial step, and most people don't even think about that step, but you must admit, it's the one first necessary step if you want to move forward and accomplish anything else using that computer. Days after my devastating phone call, as my mind finally came out of the fog of disbelief, I knew my first step was to contact Urology Associates and set up the preliminary conference with the doctor. After my first step was completed, it was time to rev up those *R*'s, dump the clutch, and get my journey headed down the road.

This preliminary conference/appointment after the diagnosis was a serious one. Dr. Cowan explained the type, the volume, and the grade of the cancer. He clarified it all: the good, the bad, and the ugly. He explained the different options available to me and the steps I had to take plus the severity of each one. He then laid out all the different treatment options in front of me. I really appreciated the time as he went through each one and explained the pros and the cons. At this point in time, I started to compile some of the information needed to make an informed decision. The doc explained what to expect with each option and also what not to expect from each option. There were risks involved for each path I could choose from, and each one involved lifelong side effects. Nevertheless, sit tall in the saddle, brother, you need to be ready to confront this and accept it. You and your family don't want to be the loser in this fight. Remember, there are risk and consequences in every decision, but try hard to make the best decision possible for you, your family, and your future, because once you make any decision, the decision now owns you.

It's advantageous for you to ask questions, take lots of notes, remember things, and find out everything you can. Also, you've got to understand the side effects with each avenue of technique you have to choose from, which initially, I have to say, will seem hugely overwhelming, disappointing, and a big psychological hurdle to pass through. But fear not. Hear them you must, because I believe even the negative information will help you in the decision-making process. Most doctors will enjoy speaking with a knowledgeable patient who asks well thought-out questions, and once again, if they don't want to listen to you, find yourself another doc, one who will respect you and will want to fight alongside you. Believe me, there are plenty.

You know, once I finished hearing about the negative side effects that accompanied each treatment option which was available to me, I started to back the truck up a little and began to wonder, is it really worth all of this? My procrastination kicked in again, and I was thinking perhaps the better thing for me to do was just sit back for a while and watch to see how things might play out. My procrastination was once again trying to push me around.

As you are reading this, I'll explain to you that I've gone through the entire process from the horrific phone call to complete recovery, and although after the surgery, I did have some of the side effects that I was informed about and told to be aware of, however, most of them have slowly faded away over the years, and the two I am dealing with have gotten less as time continues on. My belief is that, within a year, I will only be dealing with the one and last side effect. However, I'm faced with the realism that this last one may never be leaving me, and I most likely will have to deal with it the rest of my life. There is hope that it will go away too, because technology is pushing forward and hopefully somewhere in the future, there will be a cure for it, not an artificial device to help deal with it, but a concrete cure to end it. But then again, if that cure doesn't materialize, I feel that's OK, because I am alive and well. I'm a survivor and spending time with my wife. I might not be the totally all-out, happy-go-lucky guy I was before the phone call that started this journey; however, I'm alive and I'm going to enjoy the sunshine. I have a new title in my life; I'm now known as a *survivor*, and if you ask me, that's a pretty cool title. At first, hearing all the avenues, techniques, difficulties, and side effects, it is a little overwhelming, especially when we, as men, hear about the side effects we might have to deal with. They can be hard to listen to. Still, when you look at the whole picture and not just one piece, the ultimate outcome is far better than the alternative, which may be not living at all. Remember my good friend, Paul, he unfortunately found out the ultimate hard way. I certainly don't want to shock any-one reading this, but one unfortunate side effect of doing nothing may just be death. I'm sure everyone reading this, will agree with me when I say that is one particular side effect which is not a good one, bubba. Put the pedal to the metal, hold tight to the steering wheel, and rise above any procrastination. I want to be truthful in relaying my prostate cancer experience; I don't want to sugarcoat anything. This book is an account of my journey, how I perceived and lived it, and what happened along the way. This includes the good, the bad, and the unpleasant, but I do hope I can inspire you to overcome the obstacles!

I'll explain later about the side effect I live with now and will probably live with the rest of my life. But for now, let's get back to the preliminary conference with my urologist. The good doc informed me that there were different paths I could consider. There are many different techniques and procedures available, and it's important to investigate them all thoroughly. Also, all of the information I began to gather up from the doctors, from all the notes I took, the brochures and books I read, the radio programs I listened to, and the men I spoke with were now a tremendous benefit to me. All the above information became essential to me and really helped my decision-making process and should be in yours as well. My dad used to tell me to search out all the "what ifs" in any situation in order to make a wise decision—the right decision that will give you fewer regrets later. I used the "what-if scenario" in making my decision. What if I get this operation? What if I don't do it? What if try a different option? What if I don't want to go that far? What if I do the seeds? What if I speak to another doctor? What if I don't do anything at all? What if it doesn't work? Is there another option? What if I eradicate it completely along with the gland itself?

As I mentioned before, I discovered that if the cancer does, in fact, reappear at a later time, some of the techniques will not be able to be used a second time. I must stress the importance of examining each and every option available to you and not just on the surface but all the way through, like what happens in two or three years after the procedure is completed and what are my options at that point, asking your doc questions to ensure you are taking the correct path for your personal situation. Ask your doctor, "What if I do one procedure and it doesn't work, is there a second option or does the first option I choose cancel out any/all future procedures?" Do your homework.

Get yourself ready, because after this preliminary meeting with your urologist, you may feel a bit overwhelmed and a bit like "what did I get myself into." There will be many subsequent meetings, but this first one, at least for me, was a little mind numbing, but it was filled with information, facts, choices, and different ways to go. Stay focused and keep looking at your end result of being free of the monster, or you may get completely overwhelmed like I certainly did. I mean I was dazed. Keep in mind that you will have many meetings with your doc, so if you don't get all your questions out, ask them at the next meeting, and even sometimes the answer to one question will surely bring up another question. It's another reason why having a special someone with you is so important; they may pick up on something you missed. Listen to all the options the good doctor provides for you and take notes to review later. Also investigate all avenues on your own. This way, you are aware of what each option involves and the side effects also, which could possibly raise even more questions. There are a lot of options at your disposal in today's world. New technologies are changing the way surgeries are performed, and new techniques to battle this enemy are advancing rapidly, so pay attention to what's new on the horizon of treatments and cures and what they each may provide. This research will afford you the much-needed hope in your journey. New treatments are available today that weren't available to me during my time. The more you research, the more knowledgeable you will become. The more guys you speak with, the more you'll understand you're not alone. You'll gain new insight into the positive and negative side effects they experienced. Know the good and the bad.

The following list of treatment options were all available to me as I was deciding on how to proceed, and I looked at each one carefully:

Cryotherapy (cryosurgery or freezing or cold therapy). Cryotherapy destroys prostate cancer cells by freezing them; the doctor uses ultrasound imaging to place the tip of the probes in the cancerous tissue and sends a frigid minus 40-degree-Celsius gas to "hopefully" freeze and destroy the cancer. However, at my decision-making time, there were few long-term studies conducted, and I kind of shied away from this one, but that doesn't mean it's not the right one for you. Check it out for yourself.

Radioactive Seeds (radioactive seed implants, also Brachytherapy). I considered this treatment after hearing about it from a fellow I spoke with. He had it done five years before I spoke with him. He was healthy and happy with the outcome; however, after much deliberation, this one scared me a little, which is why I didn't select this path, but again, it doesn't mean it's not the correct path for others. While checking into this one, you should check out the two types—temporary and permanent. During this minimally invasive treatment, small radioactive seeds are implanted into the prostate gland to treat the cancer. Think of the seeds like little grenades that go into the cancer and blow them up.

Hormone Therapy. This involves injections each month; it may also be called "androgen deprivation therapy" or androgen suppression therapy. The goal is to reduce levels of male hormones (androgens) in the body or to stop them from affecting cancer cells. If I recall within my research correctly, I believe the androgens present in our bodies unknowingly help the cancer cells to grow, so to reduce these hormones might be a good move.

Radical Prostatectomy. This treatment involves the total surgical removal of the entire prostate gland which, in turn, also eliminates all cancer cells within the prostate which may get out of the gland at a later date and go somewhere else within my body. I chose this option because I wanted to totally eliminate the cancer that was detected and hiding inside my body. I didn't want to give it a chance to break free and wander around inside of my body, and also, I didn't want to deal with the cancer inside my body. I didn't want to treat the cancer while it was still living inside me. I wanted it out by any means possible. I wanted to silence any future threats to my life by this ugly killing machine. I was diagnosed early, which means the cancer was young and still contained in a very small area inside the gland. I was sold on the idea of totally eliminating the cancerous cells from within my body. I wanted total annihilation of all cancer cells, and unfortunately, this also meant the total annihilation of their unknowing host. Here's the thing that sold me the most on this procedure. Since the cancer was found early (very low grade) and obviously limited to only my prostate, the radical prostatectomy can cure prostate cancer. The word "cure" was what sold me.

The four options I listed above are the most notable ones that were readily available at the time I was going through all this. There was another new option coming on the scene, and its name was "cyber knife." I don't know much about this procedure, so I can't furnish any good information to you, but if it's available in your area, I would encourage you to investigate this option fully too.

I'm a little hesitant to have you read this next statement; nevertheless, I did say I wasn't going to hold back any information and I was going to tell you guys everything I knew about my journey, so here goes. There is one last cancer treatment option available, and I'll explain to you. This option is called "observation and active monitoring." In layman's terms, it basically means to "wait and see." In my own words, I would call this treatment "procrastination observation," named so after myself. I must be honest with everyone reading this book; in the very beginning of my journey, this is exactly the option I wanted to select. As the king of procrastination, I thought this option was tailor-made for me. This option lets you sit back and wait while biding your time. You still monitor all your PSA testing reports and you pay attention to what your doctor finds in every one of your yearly visits to his office, but basically "wait and see" is where you hope and pray for the best outcome while doing basically nothing, I really wanted to do this approach because I was afraid of the future, and this was a good way to postpone any action. I was frightened of the outcome, I was scared of what might be coming, I was afraid to die, and by postponing any further action, I was somehow just lengthening my time, hiding my face in the sand and hoping it would disappear. Believe me, it is a tough position to be in, so please don't think bad of me.

Now, obviously I didn't choose this wait and see option, but in my defense, I would like to say that, during this difficult time, there were a couple of things leaning heavily on me. One thing was in the past, I've lost multiple family members to this dreaded and hideous "C" word, so I was scared like most people normally would be, and I had a right to be scared because of my family history. The second, I was dazed and confused because I was being inundated with tons of information all accompanied by a ton of different choices and outcomes. So in the very beginning, the wait and see choice seemed to be a calm way for me to easily sidestep the situation that was confronting me (something all procrastinators are good at). I was told by many, including my friend Frank, that this observation method was just more of Budd's procrastination which needed to be dealt with. Also, in hindsight, I would have been postponing the inevitable, which could result in the same outcome my friend Paul experienced. Knowing what I know now, I would have been making a big mistake taking this course of action, and here's why. You see, all my PSA results were slowly but quite obviously climbing higher over the years and would obviously still continue on that upward path, a fact that was undeniable. My prostate gland was continuing to grow a little larger over the years and a little harder too, another fact that would most likely also continue on. Then came the hammer blow; I was clinically diagnosed with prostate cancer, that was also a fact, and last of all, urine flow was declining, not a lot, but nevertheless, it also was an undeniable fact. So now if you start to add all these facts together, you'd see they're not painting a sunny picture of my future. If I did indeed choose the wait and see approach, I would have kicked back and watched all those telling signs slowly get worse, not better. Those statistics have already shown me over the years what was happening to me, and it would have been insanity to think they would turn around and start going down.

The wait and see approach would have just shown me more of what I recognized was already happening. It's always difficult when you are told you have cancer, so please don't beat yourself up if you find yourself being overwhelmed; it's quite likely only natural. Take some time, maybe go away for the weekend and try to clear some air out of you head. When you get back home, take some time and begin to look over all the different decisions that are in front of you and make the right choice for yourself and all people who are concerned about you and depend on you. You know, the right choice may not be your first choice or the first idea of what you want to do. Mine wasn't. Think it through and investigate all options, and if your choice changes, then perhaps it will be for the better. I diametrically changed my choice from the easy way out, which was "wait and see," to the very tough total removal. I would like to say, total removal was a much healthier and far wiser choice for me to proceed with.

So don't worry if you do change your mind and don't take your first option.

If you have been diagnosed with prostate cancer and perhaps you do choose the observation with monitoring option (wait and see), I feel compelled to say you must also be fully aware of what you are choosing. First of all, the word "observation" indicates a passive action. You do not want to be passive at this time, my friend. I think we should change the words around. It should be called "active surveillance and monitoring option." Observation, to me, implies you sit on your butt and relax. No way, you need to diligently watch. Second, "monitoring" to me is an active word, which again means you monitor and keep up with your medical records and especially keep up with the PSA testing twice a year and any notes on what your doc tells you. Study them, track them, and recognize any subtle changes. "Wait and see" does not imply postponing indefinitely, and believe me, bud, it also doesn't mean the cancer will fade away or somehow magically disappear. The cancer is not sitting back and relaxing, it's not waiting and seeing. Believe me, it's active—very active. Its moving because it knows if it races ahead of you, its chances improve and may turn the battle in its favor. The reason I feel the cancer *knows* it must keep going is a simple reason, and here it is—once the cancer has escaped the wall of the prostate (its home) and spreads to other parts of your human body, the survival rate you may be looking at is only an average of five to ten years. That's right, the five-year survival rate among men is only at 30 percent. Now, who in the world is going to bet their life on a 30 percent chance of success. Think it through, bro.

"Find out all you can about the prostate." In other words, educate yourself about it. Some information concerning the gland is written earlier in this book, but some key questions you might think about include: What is the prostate? How big is the prostate? What does the prostate do, I mean, what are its main functions or purposes anyhow? If I can live without it, why do I have one in the first place? What makes it function? Why is it shaped like it is?

Here's a fun task to do. Ask any group of guys any one of those above questions I just rattled off to you. I'll bet you a hundred bucks that nine out of ten won't know the prostate's main function, and maybe eight out of ten won't even know where it's located. Go ahead and ask, but jot down my address so you can send me a check. Here's the thing, guys: we really need to be educated on our prostate gland. It has several small side functions which it's good at, but it has only one really big main function for being in our body, and interestingly enough, that main function also answers two of the below questions.

(1) why is it positioned where it is, inside our body and,

(2) why is it shaped like it is, like what is the donut holes purpose anyway.

Our prostate gland's main responsibility is human reproduction (that's a big responsibility). Our gland introduces the required fluids and nutrients along with our little man-made sperm (sperm is manufactured in the testicles and then sent to the prostate for processing). Once those two are together, our gland pumps them both into our urethra so they can travel together as we ejaculate them out into the world. The mixture is called "semen." This is the way I see it working. Our prostate introduces this fluid to the sperm to help in the human reproductive process and fundamentally keeps our little guys nourished during their long journey, and it helps them swim longer distances. That's pretty cool.

At this time, I would like to interject an important note. This is just another "point of interest" along the highway of my journey. This helped in my decision-making process. If any male is at the age in life where you no longer want to father offspring (and I was) or perchance it's not a goal in your life anymore to have children (which it wasn't), then our beloved walnut-sized prostate gland is basically no longer needed. We can live without our prostate because it's not a vital organ. It's required to aid in our human reproductive capabilities. I was at that important point in my life of not having kids, so in that single point, a total removal was no problem to me. Now, since the cancer had set up house and was having a party living inside my gland, then my gland had to go. That's something you may think about while deciding on what path to take. That bit of information helped me in my decision process. I wanted to totally eliminate the cancer, and to do that, I also had to eliminate his house, a house that had no more value to me. Plus, check this out, it's entirely possible that even without the existence of cancer inside the gland coupled with the natural aging process of the male body, our prostate may still grow larger, harder, and slow down our urine flow which will cause problems later in life and may have to be dealt with regardless of any cancer.

My wife and I did a lot of soul searching while trying to decide on which path to take and lots of praying too in addition to a tremendous amount of research from various sources: my doctors, many books, pamphlets, medical websites, meetings with men who had gone through this, and the world-renowned google search engine, which you can spend hours on. We even spoke with other doctors in other fields of the medical profession, not just urology doctors. I also spoke with my wife's female doctor, who simply said, "Get it out." We went through a lot of different sources of information, and each one helped us toward making a more confident decision. More information always helps and will aid you when you're ready to make your decision too. I once heard this quote: "If a man makes a decision without the information and knowledge needed to make an educated choice, it will turn foolish" After considering all the facts we could gather and also where we were in life, we felt this decision of total eradication was right for us.

Here's one very significant comment my wife made to me. "Honey, we can live with even the worst side effect because even the worst scenario would still be better than you not being here with me at all." She's so sweet and supportive. It really boosted my spirit hearing those words. I selected to have the radical prostatectomy because I wanted to permanently rid myself of all worries of it ever coming back.

I was counselled by a couple of specialists who had completed 1500+ robotic prostatectomies, and quite fortunately, these doctors headed up the most advanced program in the Denver area at the time. I felt this gave me the best chance for long-term survival. I have no regrets about the decision I made. I encourage you to research and investigate all options available to you, ask a lot of questions, and ultimately find the right path for you. It may be a different path than mine, but as long as you did your homework, did your research, and you feel confident, then proceed with a peaceful mind that you made the best decision for you, your family, and your future.

Since that ugly and menacing cancer was detected early, I was fortunate enough to be presented with a host of various treatment options which may not have been available if the cancer was detected at a later stage with more volume or even a stronger grade. Because of my family history with cancer and the fact that, at this point in my life, I no longer felt the tug of wanting children, the removal of my prostate gland was the best option. The cancer was not a part of me. It wasn't mine, it wasn't good, and I did not want it. It was not welcome on my turf. The cancer was about to be kicked out of its home and it didn't even know it, plus there was absolutely nothing the little—could do about it.

The procedure I chose was at the pinnacle of medical science and technology at the time and seemed to have the fewest long-lasting side effects, plus it was a one-day ordeal with an overnight stay in the hospital, and then you're out and back home on the road to recovery. One of the long-lasting side effects I honestly didn't even want to think about, let alone talk about, was incontinence. As it turns out, it can be quite manageable; however, to me, in the beginning stages of my journey, it seemed like a huge problem, and of course, nobody wants to have it. Now, I live with it every day, and I must say, it isn't as immense of a problem as I originally thought. I manage it quite well, and so what if I have to wear a leak-guard for a few hours a day? I'm here, I'm alive, I walk in the sunshine, and I'm enjoying life with the woman I love. Dude, it's far better than any of the alternatives I was looking at.

Remember this little Budd fact. If you have been diagnosed with prostate cancer, the longer you procrastinate and the longer you wait, the more aggressive this cancer may become, the greater the volume it can gain, and the less you can do about it later. It's not inside your prostate kicking back in a lawn chair and sipping a beer, it's like Bill Belichick and the New England Patriots; it's working on a plan to beat you at your own game. You better step up your game or you're going to lose. This is not meant to frighten anyone, but if you don't know your adversary, you are in for a surprise, because he's big, bad, ugly, and wants to kick your butt. You need to be informed of both sides of this story—your side and its side. Think for a moment at the mindset of this cancer and not just your own side of the story. You need to know the good and the bad. The good is you, the bad is the cancer. This is done to instruct you. The second important note I can pass along to you is the earlier it is dealt with, the better the long-term outcome.

Important: It takes only one (say those four words out aloud). It only takes one cancer cell to escape from the prostate gland. While confined within the prostate, it is called localized cancer. If escaped, it will be known as metastatic cancer (metastasized). Once it has escaped (spread), the cancer is free to cruise around searching for another suitable place to set up shop and hang up another sign saying, "open for business'. Now listen to this, my comrade, the cancer does not move from one shop to another shop. No, these cancerous tumors are smart business guys. It keeps the first shop up and running, the second shop is another shop all together, and now you have two places inside your body where cancer is hanging out. And this time, the place inside your body it finds and turns into a home may not be as easily detectable or even treatable. Once you have a diagnosis, start thinking in terms of self-rescue and self-preservation or, better yet, self-survival. You wouldn't set out on a three-day trek in the wilderness with just shorts and sandals—no way. You gather the necessary survival gear, boots, weather garments, fire starter, food packets. It's no different here, brother. You must think survival.

I highly recommend that you totally research every available resource at your disposal and do it with due diligence. Talking with gentlemen who have already gone through the same procedure that you are thinking about having done is a good piece of advice to hear, and listening to them really opens your eyes to new ideas. During my research, I did have one simple pleasure one afternoon meeting with an older gentleman who had a robotic prostatectomy performed on him years ago when it was in the beginning stages, and, dude, it sounded rough. He detailed for me what he went through and the fact that he was living with some side effects. He told me the best part was that he's still alive and he said, "To be able to walk in the park each day was a blessing," which means he was glad he chose the method he did. He knew others gentlemen that chose different procedures, and many of them had side effects too, different than his, not more or less, just different. Which means you should carefully choose the best procedure for you, for your lifestyle, and your future. Thankfully for me, medical technology has come a long way, and today, it's an everyday medical procedure. The research I did on this procedure detailed for me that it was a minimally invasive approach, which I liked. It uses cameras for the surgeon, which enables him a better view of what he is doing which, in turns, equals more accuracy. This procedure also uses a very highly sophisticated robot which translates the surgeon's hand movements into very detailed and accurate movements into the tight areas for the removal of the cancerous prostate. Please know I'm not advocating one method over any other. I just wanted to show you some information on all the different treatments out there for you to choose.

I had the "Da Vinci robotic laparoscopic prostatectomy," and I'm happy with the outcome, so naturally, I'm more informed about this procedure than the others, and I'm going to express my feelings, my knowledge, and information about this particular procedure more than any of the others. But listen, I'm going to repeat this over and over 'til you get it; you need to research all the different avenues available to combat this enemy and, brother, fortunately, there are many. During all your research and your exhaustive reading, you should also get some one-on-one time with men who have gone through this dark tunnel. The best suggestion I can make is for you to arrange some face-to-face meetings with gentlemen who have gone through the various techniques that are available (not just the one procedure you are thinking about). I did and it helped. One day, my wife and I arranged an early luncheon with two gentlemen. Both had different procedures completed several years earlier. I was hoping that if I could get two different minds with two different opinions about two different procedures sitting across the table from me, I might get more insight than if I met with them separately. It worked great. One had the interstitial brachytherapy seeds implanted, and the other had the Da Vinci robotic prostatectomy. I was hoping that, as we all talked together, each one might have a question for the other that I had never thought of. Fortunately, these two gentlemen knew each other, so I knew there wouldn't be any surprises for the two men, and hopefully, there wouldn't be any harsh disagreements leading to a fistfight during dessert. I had questions, questions, and more questions. They each also had questions for the other one, which I appreciated and wrote down in my notes.

During our luncheon, I quizzed these two gentlemen on the following, and if you also meet with some gentlemen, take these questions to the table and lay them out:

- What should I expect the outcome to be?
- What should I not expect the outcome to be?
- How long did each of your operations take?
- How was their recovery and how are they doing now?
- How much pain did they experience, and for how long?
- What were their side effects that I might need to get ready for?
- Did your side effects go away or are you living with some now?
- Which doctor did they select and why?
- How many doctors did they speak with before deciding on the right one?
- Did they get a second or even a third opinion?
- What hospital did they have their procedures completed?
- What helped them in making their decision.
- What were the risk then and future risks now?
- How are they dealing with those side effects now?
- Are they having difficulties?
- How many years has it been since their procedures?
- What advice do they have for me?
- Are there things that I should do or perhaps not do?

- What avenues of research did they explorer (books, internet, interviews)?
- What type of and how much experience should I look for in a doctor (e.g., how much experience has he had with the type of procedure I'm deciding to have done? Does the doc own a muscle car (just joking)?

My luncheon with these two gentlemen turned out to be extremely helpful and educated me even more on prostate cancer and the side effects. The two gentlemen gave me an enormous amount of insight and information to consider, which ultimately turned out to be one of the greatest gifts I needed in making my final decision. It was great to be able to speak with others guys who went through this journey themselves. They were willing to speak openly to me and explain the test and trials one goes through during this time. Interestingly enough, both said that, during this time, they were a little frightened of the unknown, just as I myself was, so if you are frightened also, try to take courage in the fact that it's a normal reflex. Going through the unknown is what I call "rare air," and it is unique to each individual man; however, with time, it will pass. When I met with these two gentlemen, I designed the luncheon to be held at a high-end restaurant and also started it at a good time, 10:45 a.m. This way, we could have a large percentage of our time without the busy-ness of the lunch crowd. For all their valuable information and time, I graciously picked up the entire tab. It was the least I could do for all of their knowledgeable insight. I wanted to take them out for an enjoyable meal in an enjoyable atmosphere within a nice restaurant, not at a local fast-food place or coffee shop. I tell you, the information these guys bestowed upon me was priceless! I will forever thank both for their knowledge, kindness, and time they provided during my time of difficulty. Both men stated that they made the right decision for themselves at the right time in their life. Neither one delayed the process one day longer than necessary and advised me to do likewise.

I kid you not: There are risks and side effects with any type of surgical treatment, and the one I chose is no different. It needs to be executed by a team of skilled surgeons who have the most advanced, innovating, cutting-edge programs at their disposal and coupled with an excellent care team. Even if you must travel out of state, please search out and locate the best surgeons for you at the best hospital for your care. The best doctors who perform only this type of surgery have the best patient outcomes. There will be lifelong side effects that you will have to deal with, no matter which option you choose. Each option has certain setbacks. You know the old saying, "Every rose has its thorn." Please research all options and find a team of true professionals.

This space left open for notes and/or questions you may think of:

CHAPTER 5

Surgery—Radical Prostatectomy

After a lot of deliberation, my decision for the Da Vinci radical prostatectomy was made and was moving forward. I was in high gear and picking up speed. I threw the brake pedal out the window along with the rear-view mirror because I wasn't going to stop or look back. The two principal factors which really helped stack the odds in my favor were, of course, the earliest detection possible and total removal of all cancer cells. At the time, there were three different removal procedures to choose from—perineal, retropubic, and laparoscopic, I chose laparoscopic. Always investigate if there are new choices available to you if selecting the surgical removal of the prostate gland. In fact, it would be advisable for you to look into any newly developed options no matter want treatment you choose; new ones do happen.

I went with the laparoscopic method. To be more precise, the "Da Vinci robotic laparoscopic prostatectomy." I highly recommend this procedure to any man who has selected this route. My results were outstanding, and I am back to as normal a life as anyone could hope for.

I will tell you this, and I think it's important—you should have a knowledgeable urologist. I was lucky to have one. I thank God that Dr. Cowan was there for me. I've thanked him many times with a card in the mail for dedicating his life to his profession. The urologist you typically see may not be the doctor who performs the surgery. Be sure to get to know the surgeon also and the rest of their team. Find out how many surgeries they have completed. What kind of team they have in place. Honestly, brother, it's your life, it's your survival, and your health; believe me, you have the right to know. The following questions are valuable also: What hospital will the surgery take place? How good is the hospital? How far away is the hospital? What kind of programs does the hospital have to help you now, during, and after the operation? Is this the most advanced program in the area? How many people will make up the team? How well trained are the team members? This is important too—what happens if the surgeon becomes unexpectedly ill and unavailable on the day of your surgery? What happens then? Does another surgeon take his place or will the surgery have to be postponed? You need to know. Confirm if there is a second-in-command and get informed about him. People get sick, problems arise, traffic accidents happen, so be sure there is a rock-solid backup plan in place. Find out all you can. Remember, you're the star in this program, and you are entitled to know the answers to your questions.

There are plenty of very good medical centers with highly qualified teams that specialize in urology services and the associated surgeries. Travel if you must in order to get the best care and treatment. You should be in command of what happens to you, so surround yourself with the best team you can find. Also, look for a center that has complimentary valet parking (just joking, but then again, a lot of hospitals are obtaining valet services). Search out the facilities with the most advanced program, a high-quality level of healthcare, and that maintain an impressive staff of doctors, nurses, and staff members. There are many in the world today. If something happens to one team member, you want to feel confident that another one will grab the bat and step up to the plate with no problem.

Another reason which had me look closely at the Da Vinci surgery is the fact it is minimally invasive, which translates into smaller openings or penetrations through the skin. Make no mistake though; it's still a surgery. A couple of things about the Da Vinci program I also liked—it uses high-tech cameras and an extremely sophisticated robot named "DaVinci-3D." This robot is wild and is straight out of the Star Wars movies. This robot assists the surgeon's hand movements with incredible precision and attention. You have to believe me when I say "incredible and almost unbelievable precision." Listen to this. I watched a video of this DaVinci-3D machine in action and could hardly believe what was happening, even though it was happening right in front of me. There was this normal-sized, juicy green grape sitting in the middle of a dinner plate directly in front of the robotic arms with a removed portion of the grape's outer skin (about 25 percent)! The next move was truly the amazing part and also the unbelievable part: using the robotic arms, the surgeon (while in a different room) used the computer to pick up the section of removed grape skin and placed it back onto the original grape. It was positioned perfectly in place where it had originally been removed. Again, using only the robotic arms, no human contact at all, the surgeon began using an incredibly tiny needle and thread to suture the small section of grape skin back into place, one tiny stitch at a time. Think about what I'm saying. This is a grape. We buy them at the grocery store and pop them into our mouths for a snack. That's how small this is. After all the stitches were in place and completed, the surgeon then tied a knot at the end of the stitching so the sutures could not unwind or be pulled out. The stitches were flawless and the grape was unharmed; it wasn't leaking any juice nor was it bent out of its original shape! Unbelievable! Seriously, I could have eaten the grape. A perfectly shaped grape with stitches. It looked like a miniature green football with the all laces in place. It was astonishing and totally blew me away! I had to rewind the video several times just to watch it again so I could believe what I was seeing. I would call it DaVincibelievable.

The grape thing was incredible, but when you think of the difficulty involved and the precision needed to be placing the stitches at the joining of the bladder and the urethra, you should welcome the robots' meticulous perfection and accuracy, far superior to any human touch. With this 3D robot, the chances of a human error at this crucial moment is kept at an absolute minimum. Another interesting fact that I was intrigued with and stood out to me; while using this Da Vinci 3D robot, the penetrations the surgeon has to make to enter our human bodies are obviously all much smaller than if he was going to use his own hands. Smaller openings translate into smaller scars after the surgery is completed. My small scars are only noticeable if I point them out to someone. After my surgery, I came away with five small scars; one at the umbilicus (layman's terms, the belly button), three small identical scars about 3/4-inch long and approximately six inches to either side of the umbilicus, and a very small area way off to the side. These last two small identical scars are now barely visible; however, the first scar located at the umbilicus will always be there and is still only visible if I point it out. Since I tend to think more on the positive side, I like to think a scar is not a bad thing. It's better to think of it as a flesh-and-blood medal of honor and a reminder that I was victorious over the monster that was trying to steal my life. The cancer is gone; I'm still here. So who really won? Who deserves this medal? That's right; the survivor does, and that's me. I'm here, the cancer isn't, and I can write some words of wisdom which will hopefully inspire someone, like you, to become known as a survivor too.

There are a few risks and complications with the prostatectomy worth noting, I'm sure some of the following will be complications with any procedure chosen:

Internal urine leaking. Rare and only short-term because it's fixed quickly. During the course of the procedure, the doctor performs a precision cut right through your one and only pathway the urine uses to exit the body. This pathway is called the prostatic urethra tube, and the surgeon delicately slices this in half just above the prostate gland. The top of the prostate gland is located at the lowest part of the bladder. The surgeon makes another precision cut through the urethra tube just below the prostate gland. This means two complete cuts on your one and only pipeline. After the cutting, the doctor can remove the entire prostate gland. Once removed, the surgeon must stretch this tiny tube out to make up the distance that the gland originally occupied. The doc has to make up for the newly created gap in the urethra and join the two halves together. This must be done securely because you can't afford a leak anywhere in this pipeline. Most of the time, the top of the urethra tube is stitched to the bottom of the bladder. It really doesn't matter which way it goes back together as long it does go back without a leak. Think about how difficult and technically demanding this procedure is, placing stitches at this hard-to-reach area within your pelvis region. The surgeons are good people—no, wait, they're actually extremely impressive people. Thank goodness the Da Vinci 3D Robot came along to add to their precision. Men can relate to this kind of precision; as men, we all think highly of ourselves, as we should, but deep inside, we have this caveman mentality lurking in the back of our psyche which comes out as we accomplish certain tasks. Here's an excellent example: We don't stop and move the garden hose out of our way as we are mowing the grass. No indeed. Instead, we mow the grass while getting as close as we can to that garden hose laying in the grass before we have to stop our mower and move the hose out of our way. *Wow-bam!* We messed up, got too close, and ran over a small bend in the hose with the mower and ended up shredding a section, and then it happens; reality slaps us in the face with that small voice inside our head when it shouts out, "Didn't I warn you to move that hose before mowing?" Now we have to cut out the damaged section and repair it with a splice connection only to have a small leak show up in our masterfully complete garden hose repair. Here's the point to my garden hose story—how much more difficult is it for the surgeons to repair and splice your little garden hose? Their work is understandably a thousand times more difficult. They're dealing with a reduced diameter hose within a very confined area, and I'm sure things are quite slippery, not to mention all the muck the doc is dealing with like human body fluids and other items surrounding the work area, all while trying to reconnect and splice our little exit hose. You better believe those surgeons have a stressful job—another reason you certainly want a surgeon who is far better than you are fixing that garden hose. You don't want internal urinal leakage at this stage of the game. So yes, there may be leakage with their work; however, they are very good at what they do and leakage is quite rare. It is always monitored, and if any is found, it is fixed immediately.

Bleeding. This is also a short-term effect. Bleeding strides hand in hand with any type of surgery; however, this procedure may have a little higher risk. The hospital staff monitors this at all times and always seem to be on top of things.

Secondary Hose. Oh yeah, brother, there's a small length of secondary hose which the surgeon strategically places inside your body during the surgery. One end of this hose, or I should say one end of this small diameter plastic tubing is located inside of your body right in the area where the surgeon is working, the other end is located outside your body. The outside end hangs down by your side. This second hose (tube) is a precautionary drainage device. I liken it to what's known as a "French drain" you find around the foundation of a building. This small tubing monitors any internal urinary leakage or postsurgery fluid that needs to be drained from the inside of your body. It's always good to get that excess fluid out so it does not have a chance to cause any problems. This temporary secondary tube is actually an insurance policy, because we all know the end result of that garden hose repair we talked about earlier.

The removal of this secondary hose is a whole different story all by itself! I'll tell you about it right now so I can get it out of the way, but I'll keep it short. My second tube was removed the day after the surgery just prior to my discharge from the hospital. The removal process lasted only about five minutes from start to finish. A nurse came in and explained the removal process to me in detail so I would understand what was about to happen along with the mild discomfort I might feel. She cleaned my body on the side where the tube was protruding from, and then she grabbed hold of the tube and tugged on it, removing the entire length of tube and then cleaned and bandage the area after it was out. Sounds easy. I must tell you, it was a little mind-bending to watch as this long alien object (this secondary tube) was being wrenched out from inside my body by a nurse while I was sitting on the edge of the bed. I could actually feel the tube as it moved through my body—very bizarre feeling. Watching the tube come out of my side was kind of like watching an alien space movie where you see this long alien worm like creature being pulled out of the human space traveler's body. I remember the nurse explaining that I should expect a slight bit of discomfort. She was right; there was a slight bit, and she was right about it only lasting a couple of minutes. OK, this is the mind-bending part of the story: there's only a short part of the overall length of this drainage tube sticking out the side of my body, so I didn't know how long the tube really was, and of course, no one told me how much tube was on the inside of me, so I was not expecting what my eyes were about to witness. The nurse got a good tight grip on the short piece of the tubing which was protruding from my side, and she began pulling on it. It was not a quick jerk. On the contrary, it was a very deliberate, very steady but slow pulling action. She was pulling the tube out, while I was watching. I saw this slightly bloody tube slither out of my side. It was the sight of this tube coming out of my body that was so weird and a bit gory. The hose seemed to be getting longer and longer as the nurse continued to slowly and steadily pull on it. I thought to myself, *How long is it?* To be honest, I don't know how long it was, but at the time as I was watching it, it seemed to get longer and longer just like in the alien worm movie; it was all just a little freaky to watch, and when you are watching something like this and it's coming out of your own body and it is happening right in front of you, it's blowing your mind at the same. It truly was as if it was all in slow motion at the time. I know, for the nurse, this process is normal, and she probably does it every day and it's a minor thing, but for me, not so much. Anyhow, you need to be ready for this little mind trip.

Infection. The hospital staff takes extremely good care of you, so an infection is again rare, but just in case, you will be given antibiotics both presurgery and postsurgery. Be sure to follow the instructions and take all of them. The last thing you need after going through all of this is to add another straw to the camel's back. The antibiotics are for your safety and good health. A little Budd note: It's imperative that you take care of yourself during this recovery time, but also protect yourself from anyone who may come around you who, perhaps, may have a cold or flu or coughing and sneezing. Stay away from these people and politely ask them to stay away from you. You will be quite vulnerable during this time of your journey, and again, you don't want to add to your distress level while recovering. You might want to inform any family members about this so not to hurt anyone's feelings. Try not to drink out of the same glass as others, and don't allow them drink from your glass; transferring germs will get you sick, and believe my boss, you don't need any additional discomfort for the next two weeks.

Bowel movements. Everyday bowel movements can be strange enough by themselves, but get ready for some bizarre activities in this area before your surgery. It all due to the fact that you must cleanse your system of all matter. I'm talking about the whole body's system! Plus, postsurgery bowel movements will be something else altogether strange too and may be entirely random, and I'll touch on them later; each person is a little different, but for now, it's presurgery info.

About forty-eight hours before surgery, the doctor will have you start a routine to cleanse your system. No food to start with, because you must effectively clean your entire system, and naturally, the first step would be to stop putting items in the system, and to accomplish that, you stop eating forty-eight hours before. You have to clean the stomach, the bladder, the colon, the entire digestive tract; I'm talking the whole works. Starting at your mouth and then going clean through your entire system and out the backdoor. This is a normal requirement and normal preparation method for all presurgery patients for any type of surgery. The cleansing is not painful, but it can feel strange and even a little scary at times, so let me walk you through it and help calm you. You go through this process very systematically for proper cleansing. There are several reasons for this process. However, one main reason in my particular scenario is the surgeon must flatten the colon during surgery in order to gently move it out of his way so he can perform his work. Nothing can be in the colon or it will not cooperate during surgery. I was directed not to eat any food for forty-eight hours prior to surgery, and then no consuming of any liquids for twenty-four hours prior to surgery, and finally, not even any water for the final twelve hours prior. Thinking back to that garden hose repair job, think of how difficult it would be to make the repair if the water was still running through the system while you repaired it!

I was given a set of instructions and some medicine to start my colon system cleanout, and I must say, this medicine did its job to the max! The last few bowel movements before surgery were like turning on the kitchen faucet. I barely got seated before the flow started. When you are going through this presurgery clean out and start to feel something moving on the inside, you better start moving toward the toilet, because this stuff has a mind of its own and all that stuff is looking for daylight. I changed my mind; it wasn't a flow, it was a super blast-out. You want to talk about splash-back, whoa! I have a story here about my cleanout procedure, and this is where the cleansing process got a little scary for me—the last two movements contained blood. The first of the last two movements had blood in it and turned the toilet water slightly red. It was relatively bright red, which means it was fresh blood. That started my mind riding on the proverbial emotional rollercoaster. I went back and reread the medicines instructions, and they did indeed indicate that I might see blood in the stool, and I can understand why, but those instructions failed to mention just how much blood one could expect to see or how much was normal or how much is not normal, and they didn't indicate whether I should call a doctor either. Details, people. Details! After a few moments, I took a couple of deep breaths and tried to calm my fears. I went back to the recliner to watch some football, hoping the rollercoaster ride would settle down. The next bowel movement (which was also the last movement) contained very little blood; it was really next to nothing. I managed to make it through this scary moment all by myself; hopefully now you'll know what to expect. So remember that some blood is normal and there may be some bright red toilet water. Just keep your wits about you; it's nerve-racking, but it will be OK.

Here's a Budd tip: Begin exercising your trunk/abdominal muscles and strengthen that six-pack for a couple of months prior to surgery. It will help in the days and weeks after the surgery. You see, for about seven days after the surgery, these trunk muscles will be of little help to you, and of course, the reason is pain cause by trauma in this area. The surgery does not injure or damage these muscles, but there is a lot of trauma to this area, and reasonably so. Any movement with this group of core muscles will be painful for a week and perhaps two weeks. The area around both sets of stitches (the exterior stitches you can see and also the internal ones which you can't see) will suffer trauma during your ordeal and will be painful whenever you move. The doc told me there are also a lot of nerves that run through this core area. No damage to them, just a little trauma also. After surgery, and because this whole area needs to recuperate, it will be painful to sit up from a laying down position and also trying to stand up from the sitting position. You don't realize how dependent you are on those core six-pack trunk muscles 'til some trauma is dealt to them and you need to use them for even the simplest of actions. So my advice is to do some strengthening exercises prior to surgery; it will certainly help with your recovery.

Another bit of information for you about presurgery roller-coaster rides is the preadmission meetings at the hospital! Some of these meetings can be frightening, and it is due to the amount of information you receive and have to understand plus all the legal forms with all the information you need to give. It was all a bit startling for me! You see, I was fifty-eight years of age at this time, and I never had any surgery of any kind in my life—not one. Several of the hospital personnel did tell me I should consider myself quite fortunate to travel so far in life without ever having any type of surgery. For myself, never having gone through this process before meant I was not acquainted with the detailed information the hospital administrators were required to obtain from me. Plus, I was required to completely read, understand, and sign all the forms so they knew I understood them. The mountain of legal forms might be normal for someone who had surgery before, but it was all totally new for me, and I must say, it was daunting. All the hospital legal forms obviously contain important information for the hospital to obtain, and honestly, it's also to protect themselves. The forms were in abundance, and to be safe, you have to understand each one because they are important to both parties. One form I signed stated if, for any reason, I happened to die during the procedure, the hospital would not be held responsible. That made me want to back the surgery wagon up. After wading through all these forms, I was beginning to think, *Whoa, what am I doing?* I do understand why they need this information from me, like which prescriptions I'm currently taking, any other daily medications I take, what insurance I had, my surgical history, my mental health history, my general health history, related family medical history, do I smoke, what is my average alcohol intake, any herbal supplements, drugs or vitamins I took, any illnesses I have had or my family may have had, and a hundred other little boxes to place a check mark in plus a whole host of other paperwork and information from the hospital informing me of their policies. I'm super glad I had my angel (my wife) by my side to help me in completing the forms and helped me deal with all the anxiety of everything that comes with it. Just be ready for a mountain of paperwork.

After two successful meetings with the administrators and all the forms being completed, I was able to meet a few of the hospital staff who handled the floor of the hospital where I would be completing my stay. They all came across as incredibly nice, polite, and experienced, which helped put my mind a little more at ease.

Arriving back home, it was time to start the cleanout prep work, which I mentioned earlier. I really tried to get myself mentally ready for the upcoming surgery day, but I have to tell you, when that day came, I still wasn't truly ready. Even though my stomach didn't have a single thing in it, it was still doing somersaults, especially as we entered through the front doors of the hospital.

Going through those front doors made the whole experience come to life. I felt a new since of gravity within my situation and realized the seriousness of the reason I was here. It was a big *wow* factor. My wife was right by my side, keeping me calm as she could and being supportive as always. It was quite surreal and dreamlike, almost as if it wasn't really happening to me, like I was watching it happen on a movie screen to someone else but feeling all of it. My mind had to observe and absorb every single step. I recall walking through the glass front doors and seeing the lobby open up before us. The next step—we were talking to the ladies at the front check-in desk and answering more questions while also signing in, again another step—we were gently ushered into a very well-lit waiting room with others who, like me, were waiting to be summoned by the powers-that-be for their particular surgeries. My stomach was doing somersaults, my mind was racing and my heart pumping, I knew people were speaking, but I really didn't hear them—another panicking time. I was actually beginning to calm down a bit because my name wasn't one of the names being called when, *bam*, the lady at the desk called my name and a nurse with an electronic tablet came over to me and asked my name, my birth date, and the reason I was here, checked her tablet, and placed a white wristband on me. She began to lead me through a few doors and directed me to the presurgery prep room. I wanted things to slow down and draw them out so I could think because I was unsure and nervous; again, it's rare air to me, because I had never been in this situation before.

I was in a state where things seemed to be happening more quickly than I wanted them to, and I was not the one in control. Before all this, I ran a family-owned construction company, a small auto-detailing shop, and I owned and operated a block of connected nine townhome rental units. This meant that I was always the one in control of things. I had many employees, oversaw payroll, dealt with government officials, city officials, and OSHA inspectors. Here in the hospital, I wasn't in charge of anything. I was in a state of no control. In fact, I had so little control over the situation that I found myself now standing in front of several people I never met before wearing nothing at all but a hospital gown that didn't even have a backside to it. Talk about sliding downhill. I was totally dependent on people that I had basically just met. No wonder I was so nervous. I mean, think about what I'm about to do. I'm placing my life into the hands of basically strangers, following their step-by-step instructions, and I was letting someone I barely know slice me open and remove a part of my own body. The word "nervous" doesn't even come close. However, my wife and a few of the nurses kept reassuring me that all was going to be fine, and I knew, at this point, there was no turning back. All the staff were wonderful, and in the far back reaches of my mind, I was thankful for all of their professional mannerism. My wife and I had thought it through, we performed our research well, we met with people, asked a ton of questions, absorbed a ton of information from many different resources, and the decision was made, and now, I must look forward, not back. I just had to keep telling myself that it was OK. I knew it was the right choice. I had to calm my anxieties and follow the people I entrusted with this task. The main thing that really was comforting for me was knowing my wife was right by my side the entire time, and it was so meaningful to have the one you love and who loves you holding your hand at this time—another reason you need to have someone you trust to help you through your journey too. I don't know for certain if my wife hid her anxieties and fear quite well or if I was just so twisted up in my own that I didn't notice hers. After admittance into the surgery area, the events seem to happen pretty fast. While in the presurgery staging area, different nurses came in to speak with me and assured me that I was in very competent hands. Each nurse had a different task, like placing the IV in my arm or check my pulse, and they were very busy accomplishing it. One nice thing about all the nurses— each one told me to try and relax and let them take care of me. I have to say, they did provide extremely good care. I'm so glad there are people in this world who enjoy taking care of others and make it their profession to do just that. We would all be in a world of hurt if it wasn't for wonderful people like them.

After another short period of time, the surgeon came in and went over a few key points, like what was going to happen, how they would happen, when they would happen, and he also reassured me that everything was going to be fine and I should try to relax which, I have to say, in this situation, was very difficult to do. I had to keep telling myself that I was in good hands and I made the right decision. He also reiterated the fact that they perform many of these operations and I had nothing to fear. He said it would all be over before I knew it, and I remember thinking to myself, *How could that even be possible?* Things were going fast, my mind was going fast, and I was becoming more nervous as the minutes clicked by. Things began to get a bit scary—more visits by more nurses to check vital signs. I was at that point in time where I was beginning to think I just wished it was over and I was at home again, like Dorothy in the *Wizard of Oz*, "there no place like home." The next person to come in and speak with me was the one staff member no one really hears much about— it was the anesthesiologist. He's the unsung hero in these matters and never really gets the recognition he deserves. He explained the care he would provide for me right now and also during the surgery, also importantly, during my postsurgery recovery too. Here's something funny; he is the last person I recall speaking with.

Now, we all know the surgeon is the main hero and lead man in this stage production, but this guy, the anesthesiologist, plays a very key roll. They are never listed high on the list of performers because their time on stage is relatively short. The vast majority of people do not know how important his role is. Well, you're in luck, buddy, because I'm going to tell you how important he is to the entire stage production. The anesthesiologist physician is a highly skilled medical doctor who obviously administers the before surgery anesthesia. He also monitors your heart rate, blood pressure, breathing, and blood oxygen during surgery. Then he plays a key role in being responsible for the postoperative patient assessment and care. However, because, as a patient, you are usually under the influence of the anesthesia, we don't get to see his work or him either. This doc goes through an extensive evaluation of each patient before even meeting them—the patient's past health care, current health care and any current prob- lems the patient is experiencing, and most importantly, what type of surgery the patient will be going through. He needs to make his anesthesia work for as long as the surgeon will be performing his work. No one wants his anesthesia to come up a little short. This doc pretty much tailor makes the anesthesia for each patient and determines the dose the patient receives. This doc is also responsible for the patient during the postoperative stage when you come out of surgery. Sometimes, the postoperative pain is quite severe and very intense for the patient to deal with. Imagine the pain you feel when you get a small papercut on the side of your finger or tongue when you lick an envelope; they both can cause pain. Well, an operation is like a papercut that goes four inches deep and right through the mid- dle of the abdomen—that's called real pain. The anesthesiologist is right there with you to monitor your pain level while you are coming around after the surgery has been totally completed and will assist you with your pain management. I have to tell you, my anesthesiologist did a tremendous job. I know he was right there with me because I experienced serious pain as I began to wake up after surgery. When your mind is floating around in the twilight zone and can still experience pain, you know you must be in some awful pain. I found out later that this awful pain is quite normal considering the size of that papercut. I would like to apologize to him for not thanking him for his craft, but the funny part is I do not remember his name or what he looks like, and I didn't get a chance to thank him for his work. When I was finally out of pain and waking up in my new world, he was off performing his magic for someone else. So I'm now on the other side of my operation, and the surgeon was right; it was all over before I knew it!

At this point, I would like to apologize to you all because I have nothing to tell you about the operation itself because I was *out* and have absolutely no recollection of what went on. It would be nice to insert some informative information or some enlightening words of wisdom here on what took place during the surgery, or how smoothly it went, or how many staff members help out, or even what I might have been feeling, but I got nothing for you. Let's go back to just before the operation when I spoke with the anesthesiologist. I'm lying in the hospital bed with tubes in my arm, and he's telling me to "relax," but I couldn't. He said to think of being on a tropical island sipping an iced cold drink under the shade of a beautiful palm tree. Of course, I tried to do what he was asking; however, just as I was beginning to feel happy in the imaginary sun on the imaginary sandy beach with lots of palm trees, the entire scene just disappeared. Then I had a long darkness of space. I think this was a little bit of a rip-off, because I was really beginning to enjoy the warmth of the sun on that nice sandy beach and my favorite drink in the world—iced tea. The next amount of time I can recall (it seemed very short to me) was actually hours later, when I started to wake up in the post-op area (PACU), short for "post-operative acute care unit." At this time, I had no idea where I was or what I was doing there, but I do recall the severe pain. During this very short time of consciousness, I do have a vague memory of laying down and being in an area with some curtains in front of me, very soft light, and a couple of silhouettes much like a couple of shadows at my side. One of the shadows must have been my anesthesiologist. He was there to provide postoperative care and probably realized the pain I was in and gave me some more "sleep juice" because I only recall that short duration of time of being awake and then another period of darkness, which I was told was approximately just over one more hour. When I finally began to come around, everything was still a mystery. This might sound a bit cliché, but it really did feel like I was in a thick fog and shadowy silhouettes of people were moving slowly around me. The silhouettes were my family members, and they said I was trying to speak to them but not making any sense and was mostly mumbling. After a while, the fog began to lift, and I gradually became cognizant of my surroundings. I was now in a well-lit hospital room, although I still had tubes in my arms and was still feeling some pain; however, my wonderful wife was there and once again by my side, so things were beginning to be good in Budd Town, USA.

CHAPTER 6

Postsurgery/Recovery

This chapter deals with the portion of my journey after my surgery was completed and some of the trials (rollercoaster rides) of that time. Like I stated in the last chapter, right after surgery, I was placed in the postsurgery (PACU) area for several hours for close observation and then moved into a well-lit room of my own for the rest of my stay. I spent a day and a half in the hospital which, after a little investigation, seems to be an average recovery time for this type of surgery, but I must tell you I was a little hesitant about leaving the hos pital so soon. The reason I say I was hesitant is because I had never had any type of surgery in my life ever. I had broken bones with hardened cast around them and several instances where I had many stitches, but surgery—never. This was a first for me. I truly didn't want to leave the hospital. It seemed so secure and safe to me. I really wanted to stay longer and make sure everything was going to be OK. I even told the nurses I wanted to stay. I liked the security of being at the hospital. If something went wrong, you have a host of professionals to help you. At home, it was just my wife and I. That was a little scary to think about after having this surgery done to me. During my stay, the care I received was awesome. The hospital where I had my surgery was Sky Ridge Medical Center, and they actually did have complimentary valet service. Below is a list of reasons for you to review concerning why the hospital necessitates such good care of their patients and you should expect the same also.

This first one is obvious. The staff understands you will be going through an upsetting experience mentally (I know I did). In addition to that, you will be experiencing a lot of physical pain associated with bodily trauma due to the nature of any surgery (which I was). The hospital team wants you to be relaxed prior to the surgery, and they want to do their best for you during the surgery and likewise recognize this critical time to take care of you during the post-surgery of your stay. There's a lot of things happening to you during surgery such as cameras being inserted to see inside of you, mechanical hands moving organs out of the way while also cutting various items and removing them, splicing and reconnecting taking place, but one serious item which takes place during surgery, and this one element is quite important—the surgeon will place your new friend, the wonderful Foley catheter, inside of you to aid in the healing process. This catheter begins it journey as it's inserted into the end of the penis and continues to run up through your entire male urinary system and ends up inside the bottom bowl area of your bladder. Don't ask me how this is accomplished because I was out and didn't see a thing, but I have to say, it must be quite a feat. The catheter is your lifeline (so to speak) for about seven days while everything else is healing. It keeps your urine flowing smoothly and, I might add, conveniently without interruption. It also keeps this biofluid isolated from all other organs. The hospital staff are very good at visually monitoring this for leakage and/or small amounts of blood around the entry site. Signs of blood in your urine as it flows through the catheter tube and into the collection bag are also checked. You yourself need to visually monitor this action and to be mentally ready for it because you may see some blood and possibly a few small blood clots. I certainly had seen both, and at first, it is a little nerve-racking, which began another smaller rollercoaster ride. I'm guiding you here so you don't get too nervous if you notice small amounts of blood in the tube. A little bit of blood red urine or a small clot or two is quite normal. The three points you want to look for are lots of blood for a substantial time (not normal) or blood clots getting caught in the tube and slowing down the flow and also fresh blood outside the tube at the entrance point, which is, well you know where that is, all this may be a bit troublesome. Remain calm and check often. If you do notice a lot of the three mentioned above, then it would be prudent to call the nurse, or if you are at home, call your doc's office.

The hospital team must clean and check all your surgical incisions for cleanliness. There will usually be four different sites—five if you count the drainage port site on the side. Nobody wants an infection at any of these incision points. Plus, while recovering in the hospital, you'll have a few feeding tubes connected into your wrist from a pole above your bed which feeds you several different fluids, and very importantly, they administer the pain medication through those tubes. The staff does not want any problems with these tubes or their entry ports. They certainly don't want you to remove the tubes, so don't start pulling on them! Believe me, some patients do just that. I've personally seen it happen, and it's not pretty, and it doesn't help your situation. Just behave yourself and let the hospital staff tell you what to do and what not to do, relax, and follow their lead. They will then be able to provide the best care for you.

This next one is an important reason: The hospital team checks on how much pain you are experiencing. They refer to this as your "level" of pain, and you need to learn the measuring chart for their level of pain guide. Plus, they will check to see if the pain you are experiencing is subsiding normally as expected as time goes on or if you are experiencing an increase in pain. Subsiding is good, increasing is not. The team determines what type of medication is needed and for how long. Personally, my pain level was a little higher than expected, so I was given a little extra medication but at shorter intervals. This brings me to a respectable place to stop for a moment to voice an important fact you should understand about "pain management." If you are experiencing more pain than you should be or if you think you are experiencing pain at a level which is higher than you can handle, please inform your nurse. Pain management is important, and listen up, because here's the key. It's about getting the medicine into your system before you actually need it, not after you are in agonizing pain. It's difficult for the pain meds to catch up to the bodies discomfort level. The medication needs to be in front of the pain. This is why it's called management. You need to manage your level of pain. Your body needs to be more relaxed to heal properly, and the meds help you to deal with the pain. My advice is to stay ahead of the pain. It's for your own good. By keeping ahead of the pain (or in front), you should naturally heal faster. It's simple physics. If you are uncomfortable and twisting in pain, you will not be relaxing and healing. A body needs to be more relaxed and being refreshed to help itself heal faster. Keep all this info in mind after you leave the hospital too while you are at home and taking the medications prescribed to you. Stay ahead of the pain, and don't wait until your pain level is high and you are hurting to take the meds. The pain medication takes a while to infiltrate your body's system in order to diminish the pain. That's why you take it before you feel you need it. Don't make it harder for yourself.

The hospital staff will check your oxygen level every couple of hours. Oxygen level, a.k.a. oxygen saturation. The nurses call this O-sats. Normal saturation is usually around 90 at the low end and up to a 100. Under 90 is low, and you may need an outside source like an oxygen mask. One nurse said she had seen some as low as 60. Here is a scary thought. After six minutes without air into the lungs, the human brain begins to die. A fresh supply of oxygen into your lungs on a regular basis is paramount. If you are not breathing correctly, you will not be getting the proper amount of new oxygen into your lungs. Some patients will need to be educated on the proper way to bring new air into their lungs. New oxygen in the blood stream helps in the healing process. Also, new oxygen is what keeps your lungs dry and your brain working correctly. The lack of new oxygen flowing in and out of your lungs means the moisture can't be removed fast enough, and that, my friend, is a bad thing and can be dangerous. Our red blood cells need an adequate and fresh supply of new oxygen. They are the supply vehicles for the oxygen to move around the body. The hospital staff may require you wear an oxygen nose tube or even an oxygen mask to avoid lack of oxygen. Without the proper amounts (volume of air) entering and exiting your lungs, complications can occur. Everyday air has moisture in it. Example: Set a glass of ice water on a countertop, and in a few minutes, you can watch the water droplets (moisture) in the air attach themselves to the outside of the glass. Where did you think those little water droplets come from? They don't seep through the glass. That's right, they are always in the air, we just can't see them. Although you can't see or feel them, the water droplets (moisture) that attach themselves onto the outside of an ice-cold glass tells you they are always in the air and present. If your lungs are not circulating the air properly, fluid can build up inside the lungs, and that is bad news for you, my friend. So breathe deeply and breathe often. The nurses will also check your blood pressure, your pulse rate, along with your respiratory condition. They may ask you to use a cool little device called an incentive spirometer. This is such a cool little thing to have, and it helps in the exchanging of air immensely. Nothing else comes close. Although there's a little secret to using this device, and by now, you probably know that I'm going to tell you all about its inner workings. It has been several years since I received my spirometer to use while I was recovering in the hospital, and I still have it. I still use it occasionally (maybe once a week) because it is great for the lungs, your brain, and your health. The human lungs are a mechanical wonder. They are extremely intricate and comprised of air sacs called "alveoli." The incentive spirometer really helps in getting the new air into and the old air out of the lungs. Getting the old air out and the new in helps the circulation of your blood which goes through the lungs. New oxygen in the blood is essentially important for your brain operating correctly, and this device does an excellent job at getting the blood flowing through your cranial vault. More news on the spirometer later.

Pneumatic Sequential Stockings (PSS)—a very fancy name for small air bags that fit over your lower leg calf muscles. I absolutely treasured wearing these guys and so wanted to take them home with me. They just wouldn't fit into my backpack. After surgery, and while still in the hospital bed, you may be requested to slip on one of these "PSS" devices on both of your calves which stimulate blood flow which, in turn, help prevent blood clots. Dude, that's also very important. When laying down for long periods of time and not using your lower leg muscles, you are more susceptible to blood clots; it's just the way our human bodies are built. Blood clots can be a real danger, are quite painful, and don't go away overnight. You don't want them or anything to do with them. When the nurse came into my room and placed a pair of these PSS devices on my legs for the first time, she said I would like them. Wow, was she right. I appreciated the slow rhythmic massage they provided—rather soothing, to say the least. The devices fill with air (that's the P—pneumatic) and then deflate and repeat the process over and over (that's the S—sequential) at different intervals of intensity, and they go up high over the foot and lower legs as do stockings—that's the last S. Called PSS devices, these things are great. Like getting a free massage on your lower legs for as long as you like. Once the staff placed these air stockings on me, I didn't want to take them off; it felt that good. So if you are in the hospital and the nurses place a pair of these on you, get ready for a pleasurable experience. I did see some of these devices advertised in a magazine called Hammacher Schlemmer, although it is difficult to tell if their units are equal to the same ones that I was able to use in the hospital since it was only a small picture on a page in a magazine. PS. I did familiarize myself with a less dramatic pair of these massage stockings than the hospital ones, and they are called a SCD—sequential compression device. They worked well.

After leaving the hospital, you may have to wear special leggings/stockings that support the calf muscles, because your mobility for a while will be at a low point, so a pair of tight-fitting support stockings will help to prevent pooling of the blood in the lower legs. The pooling of blood is what contributes to a blood clot being able to form, so keep those calf muscles moving please. These special support stockings are available at most pharmacies and will provide some of the same benefits as the PSS but, of course, without the wonderful air massage. (Beside the support stockings, you also need a partner to massage your calf muscles once a day to help in circulation of blood for your own safety.) The support stockings you wear at home might need to be worn for a couple of months until the danger of getting blood clots reduces, something your doc would be able to tell you. Another Budd note: Something else about these types of support stockings which would be a helpful tip for anybody. If you work in a profession where you are on your feet for long periods of time e.g. police officers, factory workers, hospital workers, construction worker, etc., it's a good idea to wear these stockings for as long as necessary. Because these support stockings compress the veins, they help reduce the blood from pooling within the lower veins and help reduce feet/leg swelling and fatigue. Check with your doctor and see what type he recommends. I wore tight-fitting, high-support socks almost daily for the years I was working on the construction site. One more kind of support stocking, my father-in-law has some Copper Fit compression socks, and he said they help a lot too.

And lastly, the hospital staff will educate you on your self-care at home after you leave the hospital and provide guidelines for you to use. It is vital that you take heed of their instructions after you leave the hospital. They care about you, and you need to care about yourself.

Of course, there may be more than the seven reasons I mentioned above, but these are pretty much the reasons I remember and I wanted to pass on to you. While you are still at the hospital, it might be a good idea to ask any questions you or your mate might have lurking around in the back of your own mind. Ask the nurse about your pain level to be sure you understand how to manage it. More importantly, ask them about things you should *not* be doing after you leave their care. For example, ask how to best to take a shower due to the catheter you are now wearing, what foods to avoid while your digestive tract is beginning to come back online, how to effectively and safely get up from a bed or chair, etc.

This next idea is mine alone and does not come from a hospital. Think about the digestive tract and the trauma it has endured over the past couple of days. It's not as if the colon has just been asleep for several days, which basically happens when you are fasting for a day. No way. Your digestive tract has had trauma and needs to come back online slowly and carefully. I've fasted many times, and my tricks are fairly simple. Start slowly and start with only liquids. Drink lots of water or any type of juice, hot tea, hot chicken broth, or tomato soup for your first day back at home. The next day, transition to heartier liquids like cream-of-chicken soup, chicken noodle soup, applesauce, or any liquid food that is not too heavy or thick for you to digest like steak, big greasy hamburgers, and hard tacos. I would recommend staying away from solids for an entire forty-eight hours because those types of foods are difficult to run through the digestive system after this type of trauma. Remember, your system has been forced to shut down for a few days, the colon has been flattened out, and things were moved around during surgery. Take it easy on that part of your body. You are going to be in some pain from what you just went through. No need to enhance your discomfort. No big hamburgers, pork chops, steaks, fried chicken, hard bread, and no really big meals. You have to use your head during this time, and your system needs to start back up slowly and calmly. The human body is not like a car where, even if you don't drive it for a week, you can still jump in the driver's seat, turn the key, and go. Everyone's body is in a vulnerable position for days after surgery. You will be in some pain from the surgery, you will be taking different medications which messes with the digestive track, and for sure, you will feel weak and tired and medicated most of the time. You'll also be wearing a catheter, and its bag will be tied to your leg. You surely don't want to add to your discomfort level by plugging up your bowel system. Believe me, brother, you don't need the kind of extra trouble!

While we are on the subject of discomfort, you will feel pain and discomfort in your core/trunk area for about a week or so. The good news is that it will subside in time. After you have arrived home from the hospital, any pain that increases daily is not normal. Slowly decreasing pain is normal. There will be some pain associated with just trying to sit down and particularly lay down. Plus, get ready for this—it will be especially painful throughout the core muscles when you need to stand up from a lying down position, so always have someone assist you with these few personal tasks for the first five days. Even just the simple act of bending over will be tough, so don't do it. Allow you helper to assist you with all your tasks. For about five to seven days postsurgery, your core muscles will be of little help. I especially needed someone to help me get up to a standing position for the first three days by placing their hand under my arm or grab my hands to help me stand up. Even after I was totally standing up, it was difficult to stand up straight and tall. I had to keep a small bent forward position while standing or more pain would happen. I really needed a helper's extra strength to get up from the bed after napping. Never be afraid to ask for help, and don't try being Mister Macho or a Neanderthal man and do something that will put yourself in jeopardy, which would nullify all the work the surgeon just completed. If you try to stand up by yourself or, worse yet, slip and fall down, you might pull too hard on some of the internal stitches, and they might tear (note to self: the doctors don't look kindly on that sort of thing). It is far better to ask for help rather than hurting yourself.

One Budd note here, and this is for your personal comfort concerning sitting down and getting up from a chair. Normal-height chair cushions are about eighteen inches off the floor and are fine if you are healthy, but because of the trauma to your trunk/core area, this eighteen inches of height causes discomfort when sitting down or getting back up. However, if you have a barstool-type chair, they will come in exceedingly handy during these seven to ten days of recovery. Most barstool-type chairs sit you higher (around twenty-four or twenty-five inches) off the floor, which means you do not have to sit all the way down or have to stand all the way back up. Like only going halfway down or up. These stools are just easier on the core muscles. Fortunately for me, our kitchen table and chairs are called "high tops" or barstool-height chairs and table, so these came in real handy for me, and perhaps you might consider borrowing one of these high chairs for the first two weeks of recovery.

I was fortunate enough to always have my wife by my side helping me move around the house and doing the little things for me which I wasn't able to accomplish alone. I truly love that girl. I have to say, it was like having an angel take care of me, plus I truly think there were other angels looking over me.

I must tell you I had a hard time laughing because of the pain within my core area. You use a lot of your midsection core muscles while laughing or, for that matter, while doing just about any type of movement, and we don't even know it. Coughing uses them. Early in my recovery, even slight coughing was incredibly painful, and get this, one afternoon, I sneezed. Oh my god, it felt like something tore inside of me, it hurt so much! One more thought. I couldn't lift a thing without experiencing minor pain, not even a gallon of milk. Again, the core muscles. Fortunately, this pain fades away as that area heals roughly one-week postsurgery or perhaps a few days longer; it's all dependent on how healthy your core muscles are in the beginning. People don't realize how much we rely on those valuable core muscles.

This pain I'm speaking about within the core is also why I've suggested earlier that you might want to strengthen those muscles for about a month before surgery. You know, just doing twenty simple leg lifts each day while sitting on the side of the bed for two weeks before surgery would help a little. As long as I'm on the subject of core muscles, I'll tell you how I keep mine in shape. I have done this trick for years even before the surgery. I lay down on the bed, on my back, so I'm looking at the ceiling, place my arms out to each side of my body. I will be using the arms for stability. Now, I lift my ankles and legs up off the bed about two feet high, I lean my legs to the left to the ten o'clock position. While still in the air, move the legs to the right side to the two o'clock position and then back to twelve and down. Easy, right? Now I just repeat the process ten times. After a couple of weeks of doing these, I advance to raising my legs a little higher and lean over a little further left to the nine o'clock and then to the three o'clock position. I occasionally go back to the earlier version of ten and two, because it works all the muscles a little different. If this seems too difficult at first, you can do this same exercise, only you start with only one of your legs at a time. One leg up and move to the ten and then to the two and down. Do the one leg 'til you feel strong enough to left both legs. Start slow and work up. You will be stronger in the core area before the surgery. This simple exercise will work all four groups at once in unison and in harmony with each other and strengthen all unlike a sit up or leg lifts alone can do. You need all groups to be strong and working together to be at maximum performance.

Core Muscles

Let's talk more about our core area muscles. These groups are not well known and are actually made up of a network of muscles.

Four large main groups, a few minor groups, and some that are in your backside, and this entire group will provide you with stability and strength. Strong core muscles will even help in preventing injury from doing everyday tasks. Let's talk about the main four, starting with the group everyone in the world knows, the celebrated six-pack, called "rectus abdominis" (*rectus*—straight, *abdominis*—abdomen). This straight set of muscles, located in front and easily seen, run vertically straight up and down your core area. Second set and visible but lesser known, the "external abdominal oblique" (oblique—slanting). The side muscle group, they start at the edge of the six-pack group and travel away from center, up your side, at a forty-five-degree slope toward your arm. Now for the two groups out of the four that are unseen and therefore less known, the "internal abdominal oblique" muscles. This group is located underneath the external abdominal oblique group and, interesting enough, also run at a forty-five-degree angle but in the opposite forty-five-degree direction, and then the one they are under, instead of up toward your arm, they run up toward your center line. Finally, the last set of the main four is called the "transverse abdominis" (a.k.a. TVA), which is located underneath all the three mentioned above and, consequently, are the deepest interior set of muscles. They wrap around your body and touch your spine. Think of it as a natural weight belt. This important group of four muscles are used anytime you move, and consequently, this is where our stability comes in, and interestingly, they run horizontally across your body (horizontal—transverse, hence their name). Here's where the magic comes in. Each set runs at a different angle than any of the others, so each one performs a different task, and working together, they do wonders such as keeping us standing up straight, erect, and tall (a.k.a. Homo erectus—upright man). Now I said all that to say this: During surgery, the surgeon must go through these core muscles to get to his intended target, so they suffer some trauma, not damage, and consequently, the effects are felt by us for a couple of weeks within our belly area. That's why we need help to get to a standing position, see how it all works together, and also why I suggested that we all strengthen those before the surgery so we can recover sooner with less pain.

Well, once again, I got a little off course, so it's back to the topic of recovery. During the first week after the surgery, not only was I was tired all the time, but just generally, I felt weak, a small difference between the two. I was taking medication for pain and antibiotics to fight any infections, so those two things, combined with the total state of weakness, made me take naps most of the time. Honestly, I would wake from a nap, try to do a few little things like wash my face and hands, run a comb through my hair, grab a hot cup of soup, brush my teeth, put on a clean T-shirt, and walk around the house for a little calf and leg exercise which, in all, would take maybe an hour of time, and after doing those few things, I would feel light-headed and weak again, so I would have to lay down and take another nap. Of course, now that I think back on this, that wasn't so bad because I love taking naps!

My personal total length of recovery time from the surgery and the trauma which came with it was about two weeks—not totally recovered just to where I knew I was feeling good again. From the day after surgery 'til my body's core muscles felt like being back to normal was about three weeks. That's almost an entire month before I was able to perform some of the very normal tasks to which I was accustomed to doing. Even at this one-month interval, I wouldn't do heavy lifting or snow shoveling, no climbing ladders, or anything of the sort. In fact, I didn't ride my sportster for four months. I must impress upon you to do the same. Take the time to heal and to heal properly. You will be better off doing it right the first time. In some cases, six weeks may not be long enough, especially if your job requires heavy lifting or climbing up ladders. I've read it's not uncommon to wait eight weeks before a person's body will be back at the 95 percent normal level after a surgery like this.

I was a construction worker most of my young life, and I can honestly state that there is no way I would have been able to return to that hard physical labor within a four-week span of recovery. I recommend to all guys to start off slow. I'd say no racquetball, no bike riding or bowling, no tennis, swimming, hot tubs, weight lifting, or even traveling until cleared by a doctor to resume such activities. Don't even drive a car for the first two weeks. Your reaction time while driving needs to be fast and strong, and you assuredly won't be. It's also not the time to paint your house or get up on the roof to work! Start slow. Start by just walking. Walking is always a great and healthy thing to do; however, remember that you might not have the strength or endurance you had prior to surgery, so start with just short walks. My first walks were out to the mailbox at the end of property and back to the front door, and that was slow and a little bit of a chore in the beginning. Walking is also great for the digestive tract, but just start slow and work your way up. A friend of mine enjoys golf and also had the same surgery I did. He did something I thought was just great. Since he lives near a small par-three course and knew the rangers that operated the course (because he played there so often), he knew they would let him walk around for some exercise. So at first, his wife drove him to the course at his two-week point into recovery, and he walked the perimeter of the putting green and back to the car and then home for a nap. After a couple of days, he walked the putting green and around the club house and then back to the car and home for a nap. He built up his length of walks 'til he was able to walk around the outside perimeter of the course and even got in some good putting-green practice! He made a small tool out of an old golf club so he would not have to bend down and pick up the golf ball. He didn't get any golf in for four months, but a par-three golf course would be a very good place to get that early and easy restart.

My wife Valerie was a godsend. She completed even the smallest tasks I asked of her during my recovery. You know, while I was at home during my recovery, I suddenly saw myself in a place where I was dependent on someone else to help me live out my daily life. It was an eye-opener, and it became an incredibly humbling experience! It made me appreciate healthcare workers even more. Valerie helped me stand up when I grew tired of laying down and get up from a sitting position, especially from the recliner chair. She had to help me up because, for me, just doing those simple tasks was difficult with the associated pain. She not only tended to me during this time, but she cleaned the house, did the cooking, washed the dishes, took out the trash, did all the laundry, and also cried with me during the tough times. Through all of this, I never once heard any complaints from her. Valerie not only completed her normal tasks around the house, but she also completed the tasks I would normally do. She did her tasks, my tasks, and took care of me; it was triple-duty for her, and I'm very appreciative and beholding. Another thing about the third week; during this recovery time, we had another wintery snowfall (about five inches), and once again, she came to the rescue and shoveled the snow from our front sidewalk. I had a thought while watching her shoveling the walkway, and that thought was my neighbors must think I was an ogre or tyrant because here I am, staying inside the warm house, standing at the window, and drinking hot tea while my wife did all the outside snow shoveling! Not one time was there even a hint of grumbling from her about the extra duty. She just stood up to the task at hand and did it all. We kept all the cards and letters from family and friends who wished me get-well messages and their support of prayers. I also have to say I received cards and prayers unexpectedly from people I had never met. They were friends of my family who had been through a similar circumstance and heard from my family about me and just wanted me to know everything would work out. Very kind of them. Prayers were being answered, and I was on the mend. It was incredible knowing so many people were praying for my health and well-being. It was quite overwhelming, but that's enough of this mushy talk. Let's get back to work.

Let's skip forward a few weeks here. My recovery was going well albeit a little slow, and to me, slow was a little worrisome, because I have always been a fast healer, and I thought I should be further along, but looking on the bright side, I was progressing and beginning to feel stronger, which is a good thing, and this really helped boost my attitude. I never was one for taking drugs or a lot of medications, so once I began to see more progress within my body, I slowed down on taking as much of the medications. The little plastic prescription bottles were almost empty anyway. I was very thankful for the different medications which the doc prescribed for me to take during my recovery process, and I also understand they are quite essential for proper recovery, so those meds did substantially help me, and I can say they probably helped me more than I possibly know, but toward the end, it is good to see the last of them. At week five, I slowly started doing some very minor yoga type stretching exercises on my own and took matters into my own hands.

All right, I'd like to provide some general do's and don'ts which, hopefully, might prove helpful to you during your recover process.

No Showering and No Bath

No showers for the first four days, and naturally, you will be instructed not to take a bath for a couple of weeks for obvious reasons. The biggest is "no tub." The reason is the process of getting in and out of the bathtub. It can be an incredibly difficult process at this time and could be risky for your stitches. Remember, you are weak at this time with little strength and also medicated, so you could lose your balance and may slip and fall, which can really be a problem. Bathtubs are notoriously known for being slippery. You may even tear the newly installed stitches. The last reason is your new little friend. You have a Foley catheter inserted in your private area, and you surely must take precautions with that along with the bag of urine strapped to your leg, and no one wants yellow bathwater. The tub idea is not so good at this time. Several places on your trunk area have new stitches which need time to heal. For the first couple of days, you might even notice a small amount of fluid oozing out of them, which is another good reason for no baths. Those are the main reasons for no baths, but no showers either. You shouldn't take a shower for the first four or five days postsurgery. Again, you have areas where stitches are, and they must close up and heal properly before a shower is allowed. The hospital staff instructed me to wait at least four days. The docs figure that, by the fourth day, the new flesh growing around the stitches would be solid enough to take the water pressure and other obstacles that a shower would throw at them, but still, a person must take caution even in the shower.

Here's another Budd note: Look at and inspect your stitches every morning. Look for "bright" redness and very soft skin, which is not good. Also, look for yellowing around the stitches (might be a pus pocket). What you should see each morning as you inspect them is a darker red color of the skin and dryer harder feeling skin around the stitches, which is a good sign of healing. After the four-day wait time, and everything is healing correctly, you can shower. Now, once you are in the shower, do not *scrub* the stitches with a mesh sponge or even a washcloth. You should, however, clean them gently, dabbing them carefully with the washcloth, warm water, and perhaps baby safe mild soap. When drying off after the shower, don't scrub the areas with the towel either, because you don't want to scrub off the newly acquired skin. Just dab them dry. After showering, check your Foley catheter, because you may need to re-tape the tube or adjust the bag attached to your lower leg. I used a couple of very long Velcro straps I purchased from Home Depot a month before surgery to help in securing the tube and bag to my leg. A little side note: Don't keep these Velcro strips too tight. Just snug enough to hold, but don't leave marks on the legs. Too tight can also lead to poor circulation in the leg, which can sometimes lead to blood clots, so pay attention to the tightness. These adjustable Velcro strips are pretty much impervious to water, so you can wear them in the shower with no difficulties and are totally adjustable. Now, for an active working individual, four days is obviously way too long to go without a shower! However, when a guy is in this situation, you must follow the doctor's instructions, and I'll tell you, it's pretty easy to go the entire four days because you are not really doing much. You are staying inside your home and mostly just sleeping, napping, and resting the whole time, so you are really not even breaking a sweat or even getting dirty enough for a shower. I always tell my friends, "I take a shower once a week whether I need it or not." That's a mighty fine joke, son.

Showers are great and good for the soul, the water in the air is refreshing as you inhale the small droplets of steam. However, when it comes to a bath, you really don't want to take a bath for several months after this surgery. I know what you are thinking for several months. Showers yes, baths no. Here's the reason. You will not be able to control when urine leaks out or the amount that might leak out. Trust me. Like I said earlier, you don't want to be sitting in your nice warm bath water, floating that plastic battleship, and start wondering why the water has a slight yellowish tint to it!

So anyway, baths are out and showers are in. Here's a new Budd hint I'll pass on to you. While in the shower, I practice what I call the "three points of contact rule." I used to preach this rule to my employees at the weekly construction safety meetings. I held weekly safety meetings with employees because they did extensive climbing of ladders with tools strapped around their waist. Also, they all climbed on metal scaffolding erected around the exterior of a building that our company would be working on, and it is still very valuable advice in this situation. While entering, exiting, and especially while in the shower, you should continuously practice to have three points of contact (stability)—two feet solidly planted on the floor, and one hand holding tightly to something secure, like the on/off water shower valve or holding tightly to the pipe coming out of the wall for the showerhead or a solid grab bar/handle mounted on the wall. A Budd guidance moment. To anyone facing an upcoming surgery, the best scenario: Before the surgery, run to the local hardware store and purchase a short ten-inch safety grab bar and securely mount it to the wall. Securely is the key word. Securely screw the handle to the studs within the wall, and do this a week or two before your surgery. After surgery, you'll be unable to install it yourself. It must be done before surgery. Better yet is to get a second grab bar and screw it to studs in the wall at the side of the toilet so you can help yourself get up and down. Another good idea is to get one of those small shower chairs and just keep it for yourself in the shower. These little shower chairs are great; they help prevent falls while in the shower. They have four rubber grab feet on the bottom of the adjustable legs so they should not slip while you are sitting on it inside a wet shower environment. One more helpful tip to pass on. Don't try to get into or out of the shower by yourself no matter how Neanderthal you are. A fall at this point would be painful to say the least and may cause damage and mess up the fine work the surgeon just performed, and the vast majority of his work you can't even see because the real work is all on the inside. Ponder this for a moment: A skilled surgeon just opened you up and cut your pipeline that carries the urine from your bladder all the way out through the tip end of your privates. That's right. Your pee-pee pipeline has just been severed in half and then stitched back together! I have done some water hose splicing at home, although that's on a very elementary scale, and if not done correctly, it will leak. Listen, brother, you don't want your vital pipeline to have a leak somewhere on the inside of you. Take care and take the necessary precautions. The only work of the surgeon which you can see are the exterior stitches. These will heal and scab over, but that takes pretty much two weeks (not to 100 percent, but close to it). It really takes about six weeks for these to heal completely. In two weeks, they will look good on the outside, and they will feel OK to you too, but don't get lulled into thinking you're all healed, because you're not. On the inside (underneath the surface, they are not), to totally heal on the inside (back to that 100 percent), you should count on six weeks. I have heard stories from some sources that stitches inside and out totally heal to a point where these areas are as normal as regular human tissue. Believe it or not, that can take up to six months.

I'd still recommend not getting in/out of the shower without someone else there to help you, even if you have installed the previously mentioned grab bars. It can be a very awkward moment, especially if you must step over the outside edge of a bathtub shower unit, and you need to help yourself and guard against accidents. Just remember to practice the "three points of contact rule." Three points = no falls. It's fairly easy to follow. Just keep two feet on solid ground and one hand holding the grab bar or shower hot water on/off handle. Now, if you are a tall guy, get a hold of the pipe at the top of the wall where the water supply pipe comes out of the wall and the shower nozzle head is attached. If you have an extra helper, let them do some of the showering work for you, like soaping up and washing the lower parts of the body—legs, calves, and feet. Remember, you will have tender core muscles for two weeks or more at this time, so your movements are slower in addition to multiple areas of stitches that you mustn't injure, and let's not forget our ever-present little friend, the catheter hose and collection bag strapped to your leg. Don't place yourself in a compromising position by bending over in a wet shower to wash your lower extremities. Get a helper. Even with a shower chair, which helps a lot, it's not an easy task to wash you lower parts.

While your helper is soaping up and washing one of your legs and foot, the "three points of contact rule" still applies. Only this time, invert the rule (turn it upside down). The three points of contact will now be one foot on solid ground and two hands holding tight (equals three points of contact). It's unsafe to have only two points of contact at any one time because of unbalance (top heavy). You will have lack of muscle control, you're physically weak, taking medication, and also, the catheter can cause you to be slightly unbalanced. Think about this, and the good Lord forbid any damage be done by any unintended quick yank on that catheter. This plastic tubing starts at the bag and runs all the way up your leg and enters into the precious tip (of you-know-where) and then continues running inside of you past the stitched area of the urethra, not stopping until it passes directly into the inside of the bladder. Please, no hard tugs on that line. That thing is a lifeline and needs to be protected with great care. Be safe and be cautious because you never know when life is going to sneak up and slap you on the side of the head.

Shoulder Pain

This is one bizarre experience and one of the weirdest pains I ever had. This bizarre pain comes not immediately after surgery, but mine came about twenty-four hours later. I was told to expect minor pain in the shoulders when this pain comes, and wouldn't you know it, just about the time I said to my wife, "I'm safe, I don't think I'm going to get that pain," *bam,* it hit me. Fortunately, it only lasted for about thirty-six hours, but I have heard stories of it lasting up to two days and in extreme cases, seventy-two hours. You see, during this type of surgery, the surgeons will pipe CO_2 gas (carbon-dioxide, an odorless and colorless gas naturally made by our mother earth) into different areas of the midsection (pelvic area and the diaphragm) of your body. This gas injection is done to help inflate the abdomen area before surgery in viewing the work area so they can have an easier time working in those areas during the operation. The vast majority of the CO_2 is released during the end of the surgery process. I have spoken with others, and for the most part, everyone has told me the same thing—the pain they feel is always felt up in their shoulders, as was mine, and also, sometimes one shoulder more the other. This has to be the strangest place for any pain to happen. No trauma or surgery came anywhere close to the shoulders, and yet, there the pain is. If you do experience this unusual pain, alternating heat and cold compress will help. Ten minutes of heat, fifteen minutes of nothing, and then ten minutes of cold, and then fifteen minutes of nothing, and then, of course, just repeat the process once every hour. I've also heard moving around will help. I've done a small bit of investigation into this matter and discovered that the pain is not the CO_2 gas leaving the body through the shoulder (like I was told by several different people). This is what I found out. The gas injected into the midsection area during the surgery really helps the doc while doing his craft; however, it causes a small amount of trauma (not damage) that is more like temporary bruising to certain nerves which happen to run within our diaphragm or midsection area. This gas inflation process can irritate the phrenic nerve, which has its origin within the diaphragm, and its endings up in our shoulders and neck. These same nerves which obtain the minor trauma within our midsection are the very same nerves that travel all the way up and into the shoulder area, and those nerves begin to ache, and the end result is pain in the shoulder. OK, that brief definition of the shoulder pain is in my own words. It might be more advantageous for you to speak with your doctor. He would most likely have a better scientific definition of how and why it happens. This unusual pain (known as referred pain) could happen to you too, so just for the sake of saving you a big surprise later, be ready for this pain; it may just happen, and believe me, you will be surprised at how weird it is.

Stitches

In the medical field, they're known as *sutures*. After a surgery such as this one, there will be several small areas on your waistline where there's a few short lines of sutures and one small area right at your belly button. These sutures are placed there in order to hold together the edges of your skin created by the surgical incision openings. More importantly, there are stitches on the inside of your abdominal area which you cannot see. Both areas need protecting, and both areas need to heal completely. If you were to harm/damage either of these areas, or worse yet, break one open, you would be in a world of hurt. A breach of the external stitches is not good but is fixable. Breaking the internal stitches could be disastrous. You probably would have to go back into the hospital and, quite possibly, go through another surgery to repair any damage caused by yourself while being careless in the shower or falling down some stairs. Worst yet, think about the damage you might cause yourself if you were unfortunately involved in an auto accident during this recovery time. My coaching to you would go like this. "Once you are safe at home from the hospital, stay at home." Board up the doors, cover up the windows if you have to, but just stay inside your place and take care of yourself for your own good. Also, if possible, don't get into a car for any reason until the day you must get the catheter removed, and then go back home and wait another week or longer if that is possible for you. The harm that might take place is simply not worth it. Think of the injury, the hassles, the loss of time, and the trauma that can be caused either by your carelessness or someone else's carelessness. The dangers are far more serious than you might think. Please pay attention to your actions and your surroundings in order to protect yourself and just hide out inside your home.

The reason I preach being careful and protective of yourself and not harming yourself is because, while recovering, we, as hard-headed men, are usually led into a false since of security. As our recovering process travels along and the pain decreases, the urge to do more will become stronger. The meds mask any pain that may still be there, and sleep time increases, so we feel better and stronger. However, we are approaching the point where the Neanderthal mind wants to get back in charge. Some might say the patient becomes "cocky." I think it's just a case of being overconfident in what we can do. One day, you do something and it works OK, so we start to branch out and do a few more or overreach, and then, *wham,* an accident occurs. A person may believe (falsely believe) that some of the off-limit things are OK to start doing again, and this is where the danger area begins to happen. This is also where the majority of accidents happen and we end up hurting ourselves. Don't allow this to happen. Be smarter than yourself, and also have your mate watch out for this period of time and have them to be conscious of your actions. A friend of mind broke a bone in his foot and had surgery with a small plate and two screws to hold things together. Two weeks after surgery, he felt like all was healing great, and it was until the Neanderthal mind took over, stretched a little too far, slipped, fell, and the rest is history. Unfortunately, recovery took twice as long as if he would have just followed the rules from start to finish. Protect yourself from yourself.

Sleeping

Because of your attached catheter and all the baggage that comes with it and the meds you will be taking, you will only be able to sleep in a limited number of positions. No tossing or flopping around in bed with this thing. One position I found to be totally out of the question for me was sleeping on my stomach, which happens to be my favorite way to fall asleep. There are only two positions available for sleeping: one is on your side, while the catheter and bag hangs tightly to your leg, and the other is on your back. Take caution, because you must protect the tubing from being pulled while you are sleeping. Believe me when I say if there's any kind of tug on that catheter tubing, it will wake you up, and there goes your good nap. There are a host of things that can pull on the tubing e.g. kids, pets, wife, and yourself moving around.

I had one special problem while in bed and sleeping, particularly while on my back, but it had nothing to do with the catheter. I was prone to unannounced aerial attacks! That's right. My wonderful soulmate, so sweet and peaceful while she is sleeping; however, there was a soundless and dangerous hazard at hand. During the night, while sleeping, I was forced to be mindful of the unexpected flopping around in the bed that my little angel next to me did. If my wife became too hot during her sleep, she would kick the covers off and throw her arm, or worse, her leg over toward me. The last thing I needed in the middle of the night was to have this aerial attack from my wife and unintentionally punch me where I had five areas of stitches trying to heal. So this is what I did. Anytime I would be lying on my back, I kept a thick pillow neatly placed on top of those precious areas. This pillow was an insurance policy. This is also something you should consider throughout the healing process; it can really help. Another item worthy of mention—children. God bless these little animals, but they may unexpectedly climb up on top of you trying to give Daddy a well-meaning hug and land on the stitches or pull on the catheter tubing. Also take caution with family pets, since many of them like to jump up and into their owners' lap. Enlighten them of the dangers and damage they might innocently cause. Take the necessary precautions and advise all family members of your delicate situation. Explain to the children why, for the next three or four weeks, there should be no jumping on the bed and especially no jumping on Daddy at any time. My advice is to let them read this section of the book—it might enlighten them—or perhaps tie them up at night—the pets, not the kids.

While we are on the subject of sleeping, you might just as well get used to the fact that you are not going to achieve a lot of real restful sleep during this early time of the recovery journey process. Two solid hours of straight sleep at any one time was a great treat for me. I kept an eye on the clock because I wanted to know how much sleep I did get, which can also be a detrimental thing, because as you begin to watch the clock, that's when it begins to move slower. I recall this one instance when I awoke, I looked at the clock to check on the time I had been asleep. It was the third day postsurgery, and I discovered I had slept for three straight hours! Man, I really thought I accomplished something since that was a new milestone in my journey. It's a mixed-up cycle of nap, take medication, nap, get up to eat something, nap, wash up and brush teeth, nap, and so on. This cycle makes you tired.

It's rather a strange time for your mind, body, and spirit. You become totally out of sync from your normal routine. As my mom would say, you become discombobulated. For me, the out of sync part lasted a good two weeks (or should I say a bad two weeks). It was several things coming together at the same time. It could have possibly been the combination of all the medications I was ingesting, which is a very common thing to happen when difference meds are mixed. I think it was the pain level I was experiencing which, again, would be totally common. Possibly may be the fact that I was constantly tired with no energy and the overall level of general discomfort that just wouldn't go away. Plus, for the first week, you can't do much of anything by yourself. I was startled at the lack of strength I could muster. I would get up from an hour nap and strive to do a couple of tasks such as washing my face, brushing my teeth, drink some more water or juice (which I did a lot of), and walk around the house to exercise my legs, take some meds, comb the hair. When done with these seemingly small tasks, I would lay back on the recliner and seriously take another nap. Even with these naps during the day and a few hours of sleep at night, I still never felt like I was getting the full restful sleep a human body need. If you combine all of the above problems with the fact I have this always-present catheter and bag strapped to my leg, I guess I would have to admit that an out-of-whack sleep schedule would be right on target and be considered the standard modus operandi of this time.

So to help aid in alleviating some of the mental worriment concerning the catheter and also with the out-of-whack sleep schedule during the night, you may want to do this next little Budd tip. I removed one of the many "J" hooks attached to the wall by our back-door which held our winter coats. I then attached the "J" hook with new small wood screws to the lower side of my wooden bedframe. This way, I could hang the measuring/collection bag along with a small length of tube onto this hook on the side of the bed and it would securely hang on that newly installed J hook during the night while I was trying to sleep. Turned out to be a bit more comfortable than having it strapped to my leg while trying to sleep, plus I think it aided me in getting a little better sleep because I wasn't concerned so much about the whereabouts of the bag and tube. You want the bag to be easily hung up and easily removed from the hook without any difficulties since you may be getting up in the darkness of night-time and heading to the kitchen for more meds. Be sure it is easily slipped off the hook. This "J" hook allowed the bag and some of the tubing to be hanging safely outside the blankets alongside of me and not attached to my lower leg while I slept—way more comfortable. The bag and tubing would not be under the covers where it might get entangled by my own movements or those pesky aerial attacks I mentioned earlier which a guy might encounter during sleep!

Now, for a few instructions on what you can do. While laying down on your bed and on your back in a comfortable and normal position, hang your hand over the side of the bed—not the entire arm, maybe just from your elbow down. You want to install the hook just where your hand would be positioned, the same position as if you were sitting up on the edge of the bed, like if you were getting up to exercise your legs or a kitchen trip at night in the dark. Now, mark that hand position on the side of the bed frame. Next move is to actually get from the laying-down position to a sitting-up position on the side of the bed just to double check the hands position at the J-hook. Have a helper hold the measuring bag down along the side of the bedframe right where your hand is resting. Test out where your hand is located; it should be very close to where your helper is holding the collection bag. This way, you can find the optimal area of the bedframe to place the J-hook. It took me a couple of tries to find the correct placement. Now, after the hook is securely mounted, make sure, while you are laying on the bed and the bag is hanging on the hook, that you have some slack in the catheter tube line. I removed the two lower straps, of the three Velcro straps on my leg, which I employed to hold the tube and bag securely to me. After removal of the two lower leg straps and laying down, I had the required slack I needed for the bag to hang on the J-hook. I still had the most valuable Velcro strap attached to my upper thigh holding the tube securely to me. The tube was securely taped to that third and most important strap so the tube couldn't slip. Frankly speaking, I never removed that third strap; it's obviously the most important strap and the last line of defense to hold the tube firmly in place and not be pulled out. The J-hook should be placed where it is best suited for your comfort while still having a little slack in the tube line and within easy reach while getting out of bed when all is dark during the night. My instructions may make it sound a little more difficult that it really is, but I'm sure you will find the correct position for your J-hook. Make sure the bag is easily slipped onto the hook. You just don't want any entanglements, and you surely don't want to be reaching too far to find it when you are half asleep on medication when it's the middle of the night and you have to get up to walk and stretch your legs or take your medicine. You need to know where that hook is located and find it quite easily just by feeling for it. Like they say in real estate, "Location, location, location." It may take a few tries to get the position right, but in the long run, this idea will come in handy.

The Foley Catheter

The catheter tube and its collection bag are both undeniably uncomfortable. First, it is coming right out of a precious part of your body, and of course, you feel every little tug which happens to pulls on it. You live with it for a week, 24/7, with no reprieve, and during that time, you have to take care of it, clean or empty. It's strapped securely to your leg, which means any tugs can be alarming. Secondly and mentally, you find yourself thinking about it all the time, and with good reason. I would find myself thinking, where is it? Is it too tight? Is it too loose? Does it need cleaning? Is there too much slack in the tube? Is the bag full? Should I empty it now? Sometimes I would think, *Be careful, Budd, you don't want the tube to catch on any obstacle!* You must be cautious not to get the tube hung up on something, which is another reason I used three different Velcro straps at different levels on my leg. I needed it to be held firmly and close to myself. I was always worried about pulling on it or having it caught on something that may cause harm to it and, in turn, harm myself. There is no real comfort zone while wearing the catheter, especially when the bag gets toward the full mark. However, let's throw out the anchor here and stop for a minute. Whenever I speak about the Foley catheter, it may sound like I'm complaining about it, but please don't think I'm complaining. Well, I guess I am complaining a little bit, but really, on the positive side, I'm thankful for this device and thank God for Frederic (the man who came up with this idea). Without this wonderful little device, believe me, life at this time would be a very unpleasant experience. The catheter makes the recovery process far more bearable than it could ever be, and I must admit, the thing is rather convenient. You have to learn a little bit about catheters and be able to work around all their little complexities that come with this nifty unit.

One fact about the "Foley" catheter (Foley is the technical name for the type of catheter I was equipped with, and it's the most common type of indwelling urinary catheter. Named after Mr. Frederic Foley, who design it way back in 1929), it's not always an automatic draining device, although it might be considered as one. There are no moving parts and no mechanical workings, no batteries, and no cord to plug in because for this device to operate, it gets all its power from gravity. During the twelve days I was equipped with the Foley catheter while sleeping or napping, I would sometimes wake up with an urge to urinate, and of course, with this catheter thing attached to my body, all I had to do was just stand upright. That's the simplistic beauty of this thing, and it's undeniably great. When the urge to urinate starts knocking, guess what? That's right, all I had to do was remove the covers, get out of bed, and stand upright. I was even able to leave the bag on the hook. *Wow*, it was kind of cool to feel and see my body working efficiently and smoothly in conjunction with the catheter without my mind handing out any instructions. I didn't have to walk the distance from bed to the throne room and no turning on lights while your eyes are used to the dark. I would just stand up, and the physics of gravity would go to work for me. Everything did its proper job, my body and the catheter worked as one unit, and I just watched the fluids make their journey from inside of me, through the tube, and down to the measuring pouch. I watched it all work. It was so strange to go through all the motions without actually going through all the motions. You need to be aware of this process and how the catheter works because you need to monitor what is happening and when it's happening for safety reasons. Your duty is to make sure there are no leaks or kinks on the outside and no obstructions on the inside of the tube e.g. a blood clot. A blood clot may happen. You won't feel it, so you must look at the tube carefully. I was instructed by the nurse to observe the fluids as they traveled down the clear tube and into the bag and look specifically for clots or blood. A few small blood clots are normal, so if you see a few and they are small, there should be no need for alarm; that is common and normal. Small clots will easily flow through the tube, sort of like a raindrop making its way to the ground, because it will be smaller than the inside diameter of the tube. A large clot, on the other hand, will be obvious because it will be the same diameter as the tube as it travels through and may even get stuck, like at the location of the Velcro strap, because at that location, the inside diameter of the tube will be a little smaller. That's why you observe the operation or the motion of the fluids. My experience while wearing Mr. Foley wasn't too hectic. A few close calls, but all in all, it went well. I observed several small clots at different times and only one that I would have classified as a large clot, but still, they all made their own way through the tube and into the holding bag without any problems. The clot held together and strangely did not tint the color of the urine. When you first see a blood clot, it will be a little alarming. However, just hold on; it's one of the reasons you're reading this book—to be informed. Just watch the clot and make sure it travels the length of the tube and into the bag. The anxiety, the panic, and the rollercoaster ride of fear will pass just like the clot will surely pass. It's only when large and multiple clots are present and the color of urine changes to red (which indicates blood) and perhaps you have some pain occurring—that's when you should be alarmed. I would recommend calling the doc about that situation to be on the safe side.

The Foley catheter is going to be your friend for a while, so you might as well make an easy go of it. You may experience a little pain at first, and maybe at the exit point, and you surely know where that is, but most pain dissipates slowly within the next couple days. You will also have to get used to the feeling or, should I say, the sensation of having to urinate often. This urge will come because of the new and unusual pressure inside the bladder. In my opinion, I think the pressure is cause by the funnel-shaped water balloon device that is located at the top end of the catheter tube which is now resting on the bottom area inside the bladder. This funnel-shaped balloon is what keeps the tube from being pulled out (very important); however, it also puts pressure on the bottom of your bladder, which may simulate to the brain the need to urinate. I had very little pain associated with wearing the catheter through the twelve long days of it being attached to me. Actually, twelve days is at the long end of the timeframe; seven days seems to be normal. I was also advised by my doc that I may experience what doctors called "bladder spasms," but I can't give you any information on bladder spasms because I never had any. So you are going to have to ask your doc about them. I think the spasms may be related to the funnel-shaped balloon also, but fortunately for me, those spasms never developed, which was another Amen moment!

Here's a good place to stop and tell a short story about myself while I was at home, recouping and wearing my new little sidekick, Mr. Foley D. Catheter, and why I wore it for twelve days instead of the normal seven days. There were a series of unfortunate and peculiar events that came together to make this story happen. First off, I arrived home from the hospital to begin my recovery, and day one went as well as good be expected. A little painful at the tip of my you-know-what where the tube was exiting, and I was quite sleepy and tired most of the time, and my core muscles were of no help. I guess you could say everything was going according to plan until the following day when I did have a rocky moment. I went into the bathroom to comb and wash up. I caught the catheter tube on the bathroom lower cabinet door handle. *Ouch!* No fun. I wanted to protect the tube, but I couldn't wear my Levi's jeans with this thing strapped to my leg; however, my wife dug out my old and long bathrobe and I put it on. It was so comfortable and easy to wear. It was large for me, floor length, and came with a hoodie too. This robe was something that you might see Gandalf wearing. I wore nothing but that robe for the next four days. As the pain was lessening, I thought about a pair of baggy sweatpants I had in the back of the closet I never really wore because they were way too big for me, but now, I was thankful to have them. They were easy to slip over all the tubing and bag. A floor-length robe and large pair of oversized sweat pants might be a good idea for you to get before the surgery date.

As the days slowly passed, it was on day five and approaching forty-eight hours to go before Mr. Foley was scheduled for extraction. This was when things took a turn for the worse. I was back in my robe and sipping my usual morning cup of hot spiced orange pekoe and black tea. While enjoying my tea and standing at our front window, I was looking out and up toward the sky. I noticed some dark, ominous-looking clouds forming, which were now beginning to block out the sunshine trying to come through and there was that certain rocky mountain chill in the air. Just prior to making my tea, the television weather forecaster predicted snow later in the day but nothing too serious. I mean, it is January in Colorado, and we get lots snow and cold this time of year, so nothing was out of the ordinary and didn't set off any red flags. *Wow*, did the weather forecasters blow this call! Wait, don't jump ahead of me.

About three hours later, I woke up from a nap and I made a second cup of tea. I wandered over to the same front window, and sure enough, it was indeed beginning to snow, just like the forecasters forecasted. It was one of those magical moments when you look through the glass window to the outside world and start watching the multitude of little fluffy white snowflakes falling so innocently and silently. It makes you think that Nature looks so beautiful; the pure white fun-loving snowflakes slowly tumbling over each other as it actually appeared as though they're having fun floating down from the sky and almost bouncing as they hit the ground. I kind of felt like I was a kid and I was inside a Walt Disney snow globe.

Throughout the entire day, the snow continued to fall. At first, there was no accumulation of snow. In fact, it really melted into the grass and sidewalks as the snow turned into damp ground. Well, as more time passed and the temperature dropped, the snow now began to cover the grass areas. Just an hour later, it was beginning to cover the sidewalks and accumulate on the streets too. My outside world was beginning to turn snowy white, yet it stilled appeared to be a normal Rocky Mountain light snowfall and not a hint of what was to come.

Ah, the story continues. It's now late in the evening, and thirty-six hours before extraction, and my outside world is white with snow, even on the trees and rooftops. I turned up the furnace as I started to prepare for, hopefully, a few hours of good sleep, but I must tell you, I was beginning to worry just a little bit about this snowfall. I was born, raised, and still live in Colorado (a second-generation native, which is rare), so I know what can happen within our weather system.

Anyhow, during the night, I had my normal "sleep, wake up, sleep, take meds, sleep, wake up" nighttime routine, and after getting out of bed in the morning, I cruised into the kitchen and made that morning cup of hot loving tea. With tea in hand, I moved to the same window and pulled the curtains back so I could look out and see my world. *BAM!* What a surprising difference. Those little fun-loving snowflakes weren't as fun-loving any longer, and I began to think, *Dorothy, we're not in Kansas anymore.* In fact, it was obvious that the snow fell unceasingly throughout the night. Snow covered everything—the grass areas, the trees, rooftops, sidewalks, streets, cars, nothing was escaping the snow, and in fact, at this particular time, it was already about five-inches deep. Again, five inches in Colorado is manageable, but no forecaster was predicting this one correctly. Those cute little snowflakes we were so fond of yesterday weren't so cute this morning, and they certainly weren't very little either. They were much larger now and coming down considerably faster. It appeared as though all the snowflakes, sometime during the night, joined forces with Darth Vader and were in some sort of angry attack mode against my friendly empire! My neighbor's tree limbs were not only bending because of the weight of the snow, but one actually broke and was hanging straight down. My first thought was a rollercoaster ride, and then my second thought was, *OK, Budd, relax a little bit. We don't need one of those rides. We're almost through this. Only hours away.* I was concerned about my catheter extraction. It was scheduled for 10:00 a.m. the following morning. Now, if the snow would stop, everything would work in my favor and be fine. So I took my own advice and stared to relax while sipping the tea, but in the back of my head, I was a little worried. My extraction was only twenty-four hours from this point, and the cards being dealt on the table weren't looking too favorable for me to win this hand. I was just hoping it would slow down and stop. No such luck. Snow fell all that day, and the wind picked up while the snow piled up. By 10:00 p.m. in the evening, the snow was still falling, and now, it was only twelve hours before my appointment. Road closures were starting to be announced on the late news. About eight inches of snow was now on the ground with no apparent signs of letting up. This was a big-time snowstorm in the Rocky Mountains, and the big-time weather forecasters were now upgrading this storm to a Colorado blizzard warning! It was kind of an eerie feeling. It was cold and dark outside, and the wind was howling. I couldn't see any headlights because no cars were moving. Believe me, nothing was stirring, not even a mouse.

When I awoke the next morning, I arose with such a clatter. I quickly ran to the window and threw open the sash to view what the storm had left. Well, first of all, I really did arise early, but with my catheter in place, I couldn't really run quickly to the window, and there isn't any sash on my windows. However, when I did look through the window to the outside world, it was a complete and total white out. That's one large red flag of concern. I knew, without a doubt, this was not the ideal situation to be in.

I made my way to the phone and placed a call to the doc's office, just checking on my appointment for the Foley extraction this morning at 10:00 a.m. Well, here's another point of the story that went wrong. I called, and the phone service answered. Another red flag. No nurses, only a phone service. Well, the phone service told me no personnel were in the office, they're not coming into the office, and all appointments were cancelled for today and possibly tomorrow also. She then told me not to expect anyone until the storm was over and the staff could make their way on the roads. OK, now I'm a reasonable individual, and I couldn't blame the doctor or his staff for not making it. This storm turned out to be a wicked one, and as I pondered my own situation, honestly, I began to feel a little relieved (you know, look for the good in things). I honestly didn't want to climb into the truck and try to navigate my way through the weather in a Colorado snowstorm with this catheter strapped to my leg and the tube running through my exit pipe. Wouldn't that be a lot of fun? Just think of me and my wife driving on icy and snow-filled roads, possibly having an accident with this thing strapped to my leg. What if it started to freeze? Needless to say, we just stayed home and made a bunch more tea which, consequently, filled my bag up faster. About a foot of snow on that faithful day! Well, the storm continued for another twenty-four hours, although you could see it was slowing down considerably. It was quite apparent that I wasn't going anywhere and also that I would be wearing this catheter for a while longer. It was a heavyweight snowstorm, lots of bad roads, lost time, and a backlog of patient appointments at the doc's office. After the storm was finished and I finally connected with the doctor's office staff nurses, I was told my extraction of Mr. Foley was pushed back five more days than the originally scheduled date. I now had a few more days to frolic around with Mr. Catheter. Yeah, loads of fun and end of story. Sorry my story was so long, but hopefully, you came away with a few laughs, and the real meaning of the story is that, during your journey, things will not go as planned and it may not be anyone's fault.

There's one more little note of interest I'd like to pass on to you. Again, I didn't have this nugget explained to me. I wish I would have been told. I found out the hard way, all by myself, but I'm here to help you with nuggets of information so your journey will be smoother, so here goes. About twenty-four hours before your doctor visit for your extraction of the catheter, I suggest you deliberately slow down on your fluid intake, drop down to around forty ounces, and here's the reason why. While wearing the Foley catheter, you may drink all you want because the catheter does the work for you. I mean the fluids go right through you, almost like they don't stop anywhere on their trip through your body. However, after the removal is completed, you are now back to doing all the work yourself, and at first, it's not easy. So to help yourself out a little bit, it is a good idea to lower the intake at least twenty-four hours before and several days after, or even perhaps a week after the extraction. It might be even longer like mine was. It all depends on your own personal situation. After my extraction, it was horrendous, all because I didn't slow down on the amount of liquid intake; it was a total mess. Please don't make the same mistake I did.

My Foley extraction day finally came (day twelve). Extractions are done within your doctor's office, not at a hospital. Quite convenient. I'll explain how an extraction is completed. As I sat in the exam room, my other doctor, who is Mr. Jeffery, came in and sat down with me. Jeffery was the one who did my extraction, and this was how he started. He said, "Now, Mr. Nielsen, trust me, this is a very simple procedure and goes quickly." He told me that I might feel some mild discomfort with the removal. I have to say, Jeffery's mild and my mild were on two different scales; however, on the other hand, Jeffery was correct. It was a fairly simple procedure. From the time I entered the catheter extraction room until I was leaving, it was approximately twenty minutes. That also included our discussion about the storm. Out of those twenty minutes, the actual extraction was close to only five minutes and the time it takes to pull out the tube was only ten seconds. Simple, or so it sounds. Just wait a minute. Don't get ahead of me.

Actually, Mr. Jeffery is a jolly dude and pretty cool. He totally described the extraction process to me in detail so I would be ready and aware of all the action and the mild discomfort that goes along with it. He told me just what he was going to do and how he was going to do it. Jeffery wanted me to be mentally ready because, once it starts, it has to go all the way; there's no stopping in the middle for coffee and donuts. Once he was convinced I was ready, we started. He explained to me about the funnel-shaped balloon the surgeon places inside my bladder during the surgery. The key thing about this balloon—it's in there to take all the abuse while your body heals. It's only temporary, but it safely holds the catheter in place so nothing pulls it out. The funnel balloon sits inside the bladder at the lowest point. Because of the balloons position inside the bladder, it will give you the feeling of a full bladder, which makes you feel like you need to urinate most of the time you have it. This funnel device is tightly connected to and holds the catheter tube in place. Jeffery's first job was to educate me on how he was going to extract this device, which he certainly did. Jeffery's second job was to deflate the funnel-shaped balloon in order to decrease its size and diameter so it becomes small enough to be removed along with the tube through the entire length of the urethra system, from bladder on down, and the whole thing would come shooting out the end of my personals. Doesn't that sound like a party? Brother, let's just stop here and think about those words for a moment. Just contemplate what is about to happen to me.

OK, Jeffery deflated the balloon device and waited a minute to ensure it had enough time to shrink down to its smallest diameter size possible. He said he would now grab hold of the tube which was dangling out of the end of my you-know-what. His third job was to give the tube a very steady but clean pull and take out the entire length with no stopping until the complete entity came out with no problems. Again, brother, no guy in the world can ever really be ready for this kind of maneuver, and I was no exception. I had this tube connected to me now for twelve long days and nights, and I truly wanted to part ways with it, and this extraction had to be done, and my time was up. So I looked at him and said, "Sounds simple enough. Let's do it." Even as those words left my lips, I couldn't believe I just said what I said. I was also a little skeptical on the mild discomfort we discussed earlier. We have to stop for a second right here before we continue any further. The good doc Jeffery also gave me a verbal sentence which I needed to commit to memory so I could repeat it back to him out loud while he tugged and extracted the entire length of the catheter tube and the now-deflated funnel balloon. He suddenly stopped, turned his gaze straight at me, and this time, he wasn't smiling.

He looked me straight in the eye and suddenly took on a very serious side when he said, "Timing is crucial now. Once I start the extraction, there can be no stopping. It must come all the way out, and it should be a clean one-step process." So this is how it went down. As I would start speaking my memorized sentence, he would start the extraction procedure. When I was in the middle of my sentence, he would be halfway through the extraction. When I got to the last word in my sentence, he would be at the last part of the extraction, which is where the funnel-shaped balloon would be firing out the end of my little private part. It sounded like a good rock-solid plan of attack to me.

The sentence Jeffery had me repeat out loud while he was completing the extraction was, in reality, a diversionary distraction technique he used so I would be focused on and thinking about the words I was speaking and not on what he was doing. It actually worked quite well. I started speaking, and he started pulling. Half way through, I began feeling the discomfort, which wasn't so mild; however, by the time I got to the last few words of the sentence, I was literally screaming them out loud because of the discomfort! Everyone on the entire staff and I bet half the patients in the waiting room heard me scream too. Jeffery, being cool, just leaned back and laughed loudly like he was jolly Santa Claus and he just gave me a big present. This time, I was right; it was more than mild discomfort, but Jeffery was also right. It was simple, quick, and my discomfort only hurt for a couple of minutes and then began to subside. I have to say I was quite happy to be disengaged from the catheter and have one more part of my journey behind me. The catheter was an especially good thing to be looking at in the rearview mirror. I lived twenty-four hours a day for twelve days with the catheter. To say I was happy it was over would be an understatement. Medical technology is a wonderful thing, and thank God for it, but being done with the catheter really did put a smile on my face. Now, this may sound funny but, I felt like I had a new sense of freedom. I could walk normal again. It was a lot like letting a dog off his leash so he can run free in the park. This was just one more milestone along the journey, it went well, and it was now over. I had a smile on my face a mile wide.

While on the subject of the Foley catheter, allow me to elaborate on a few things.

1) The downsides. This thing is cumbersome, sometimes embarrassing, needs emptying every couple of hours (it was for me, I drink a lot of fluids) and, for obvious reasons, is uncomfortable.

2) The upside is it is wonderfully innovative and works amazingly well. It is immeasurably needed. I don't understand how anyone would go through this procedure and not have one of these devices.

So if you add all the different factors into the equation, all of these downsides and the upsides and then subtract out all the misery everyone would have to endure if we did not have it, the total would show even the downsides turned into good sides after all.

Another Budd tip: While you're wearing one of the Foley catheters, you must understand personal hygiene is essential, particularly at the point of entry. I took certain precautionary measures while wearing mine, and I'll pass them on to you.

First: Cleaners. Every even-numbered day, I used a cotton ball dampened with rubbing alcohol (91 percent isopropyl alcohol) to clean the area where the tube entered my body and then used a sheet of paper towel with more rubbing alcohol to clean the entire length of tubing, including the outside of the holding bag. I used the 91 percent isopropyl alcohol first and then a small amount of hydrogen peroxide on a different cotton ball to again cleanse the area where the tube entered my body. I always used the rubbing alcohol first because it evaporates quickly followed by the hydrogen peroxide, which doesn't evaporates quickly. The rubbing alcohol has antibacterial properties and is also known as an astringent. Alcohol is better at removing oils than the hydrogen is. Hydrogen peroxide is a sanitizer and disinfectant, and the two are very close to each other in what the can do; however, they are a world apart in their chemical makeup. Using these dual-duty cleansing products is my own idea. It did not come from any hospital staff or doctors. There is a whole world of debate over whether to use these products in tandem, but I like their dual and complimentary personalities. I've used them together for years, and they work well for me. I use them in conjunction with each other for many things—cuts, scratches, splinters, etc. Carefully read the labels, do some extra research, and decide for yourself.

Second: Every odd-numbered day, I used a handy antibacterial wipe with an extra moisturizing ingredient which counters any drying effects the previous two cleaners may have. I found the wipes at Target (Up & Up Antibacterial Wipes is their label). They claim to kill 99 percent of germs and are very mild. I used them to clean all of my personal areas. You know the ones—Mister double-O and seven. I even cleaned the entire catheter hose and the outside of the bag with these wipes. It is very important to keep all areas clean and sanitary. A smaller Budd note: If you begin to feel discomfort at the tip of your penis right where the tube enters it, a very small dab of Vaseline jelly at the point of entry will work wonders to soothe this area.

Two more very good cleansing products I would like to clue you in on; however, I couldn't find these two items at a regular store. You must go to a medical supply store to purchase these. One I discovered is a cleansing foam I use in the shower and, I have to say, works quite well and helps you feel cleaner than regular soap. It's produced by "Convatec." It is a high-foaming, non-aerosol, pH-balanced cleanser. It is made to clean and dissolve any type of fecal matter which may be caused by incontinence or anything else for that matter (www.convatec.com). This product cleans all areas squeaky clean, and it contains aloe vera for soothing action, which I happen to like. I use this cleanser in place of my ordinary soap for the areas impacted by the use of my catheter. The other cleanser is called "Phytoplex" by the Medline company. I highly recommend getting both the wipes and cleanser to clean all your personal areas while wearing the catheter and even after it is removed. These cleansers work so well that, even though I am five years out from my surgery, I still use the Convatec cleansing foam once a week.

I was a happy, no-worry kind of child as I was growing up, but as I was turning older and into a man while working with my dad in the business, the worriment and concerns of the work-a-day world began to enter my life, which is only natural in the hectic lifestyle everyone lives in today. But during this prostate cancer journey, I don't think I was worried about so many different things happening to me, my body, and my life at any one time previous to this. My journey put my mind through so many different changes, and my body too. It was definitely one emotional rollercoaster life-changing ride. I'm not sure even Bilbo Baggins or Frodo carrying the ring went through this much! I would start to freak out about some of the difficult decisions I was going to have to make and someone would help me out. After a while, I would start to freak out about the different experiences I would have to go through, but help came. I would begin worrying about another problem I was experiencing, and as I was in the midst of trying to solve it, another one would crop up, and then someone would reassure me that all was quite normal for what I was going through, so I would try and calm down only to find something else would arise, and once again, the rollercoaster ride would start all over. One example. After surgery, my GI tract wasn't working correctly, which just started me on another wild ride, which is a great segue to the next paragraph.

GI Tract

One thing I did sweat over, was how to start up my GI tract after such a lengthy time with no food traveling through it and the surgery process which flatten it out greatly. My grandfather taught me how to abstain from food (fasting) for a period of time (one to three days) to help clean out my body, plus he told me how to properly start the system back up again after fasting. Even with his excellent advice in my head for guidance, the thought of starting up my system after this operation, coupled with the shutdown process I went through prior to the surgery and also the flattening out during surgery, was a little scary for me and I was nervous, but I had a right to be very apprehensive, I tell you why latter. I stopped having any bowel movements sixteen hours prior to surgery and it was 96 hours after surgery before I finally had my first bowel movement. That's a long time. Toward the end of the 96 hours I was truly sweating bullets, rollercoaster ride. I mean, for years I have been as regular as clock-work and this may be too much information for most people to hear, but you know I'm going to tell you anyway, there's no need being modest now; it's what this book is about. Before surgery my GI system was regular, it's like I was a human Timex clock—once a day every morning somewhere between getting out of bed and before 9:00 a.m., I was in the throne room doing my "daily constitutional." So for me and my system to be out of service this long was truly worrisome. Plus, factoring in the way I had to force my body's system to shut down before surgery, adding in all the different medications (which always messes with the GI track), the entire surgery process where they move everything around or out of their way, all the trauma to my insides, and the many days without any bowel movements, believe me—it was far more than just bothersome. Thoughts were flying through my mind of a flattened intestine that would not come back to life. A flat or plugged-up colon can be a real problem! Budd's rollercoaster ride started again. Toward the end of the 96 hours, I was scared, nothing was moving. I was close to calling the doctor. In fact, I did call the on-call number, which I was provided with postsurgery, about 50 hours into the no bowel movement period. The assistant assured me it was all quite normal and she calmly explained that I should only have very soft food for the first couple of days so that the colon could start back up gently and slowly, but it should have no trouble starting back up, she reassured me that the human body is resilient and will start, just takes time.

A few things were working against me here. All the different medications I was ingesting, they always play a part in slowing down the digestive track, the presurgery cleanout routine with the enemas to clean you totally out, and then the colon flattening during surgery so the doctor can move it out of his way while working in the area. They were all causing me a gang of worriment. Correspondingly, I think this flattening out of the colon was my biggest worriment, and as I said earlier, I had a very good reason to be worried. You see, as an infant, I was dealt a serious blow, a very serious health problem which lasted until I was around thirteen years of age. I had a minor kink in my bowels a.k.a. a partial twisted bowel, painful to endure as a child, not twisted enough for surgery but could be controlled with diet, and the doctors told my parents that this small kink in the child should be outgrown as the child grows. Nevertheless, my childhood diet of mostly liquids, high-fiber food, and the food I did eat I was instructed to chew thoroughly and completely, lots of water, even hot tea, and a half-glass of good old prune juice every other day really helped me out during those childhood years.

(Hey, while writing this, I just had an illuminating realization, an epiphany if you will. I think it's a carryover from my childhood. Maybe that's why I drink so much water now plus maybe my love for tea also. Very interesting).

As I was growing up, this twisted bowel thing was difficult for me. Not only was it very painful at times, but it restricted my diet, which is never fun for a child, because as a kid, you want to eat everything in sight. Plus, I would occasionally get so plugged up my folks would have to administer enemas to me in the bathroom a couple times a month because I would eat something I wasn't supposed to eat and had to get help in getting it all cleared out. I probably had twenty-plus enemas a year. So I hope you can sympathize with me, because at this particular time in my journey, all those nasty memories from my childhood were flooding back in and I really didn't want to return to an enema every week. That started another rollercoaster ride. All these things, both pre- and postsurgery cleaned me out so well that it actually is taking a bit longer to start back up. This was far longer and more serious than the simple fasting I was accustomed to. I was very cautious about introducing solid food back into my system. I started with only liquids like hot clear soup. Seriously, I had only chicken broth and fruit juices—no solid food of any kind. I was that worried. It was only on the third day I began to introduce soft foods like yogurt, pudding, Jell-O, and some very runny oatmeal (which is the way I enjoy it), and then small amounts of small-curd cottage cheese, and then moving onto breakfast cereal and toast. That, my friend, is what you call, extremely cautious.

An important thought worth inserting here. A person must chew all food extremely well. The more you chew your food, the better your teeth will puree and grind the food into smaller bits. The smaller the food bits, the easier the body can further break it down, and the easier it is to travel painlessly through your entire system. Both your mouth and teeth work in conjunction with each other, much like a countertop blender does. The blender will chop or turn food into mush. I learned in a cooking class once that mushed or pureed food is better for the digestive tract because it can absorb more of the nutrients from the food we consume. The body does not have to work as hard to break down the food if you break it down beforehand. Simple physics. The more you break it down, the less work for the digestive tract to perform. I also found out this is why some folks may not get a good night sleep. When you eat a big meal at night and

136

don't chew your food really well, your insides are working all night trying to break down the late-night meal. Consequently, you may wake up the next day feeling tired as if you didn't get enough sleep. Well, your body didn't get enough sleep, that's why, because while your head may have been sleeping, your body was working for hours on digesting all of that late-night food.

In retrospect, I sort of prolonged the length of time my system took to come back online, because I must admit that I was apprehensive and worried. I knew the docs had to flattened it so they could perform their magic, and I was concerned that my colon wouldn't inflate back to normal size and normal shape, or worse yet, they may inadvertently create another kink within my system, which might just cause me more problems in the future. But I had a good reason to worry about this happening because of the problems I had as a kid. I had to be careful what I ate or I suffered the consequences. Having countless enemas to help you go to the bathroom when you are a little boy is not fun. After the surgery, my colon did indeed inflate to its normal size; it just took a while, and fortunately, there were no long-lasting side effects. Amen to that. It just took a bit longer to come back; hopefully, you can now understand my worriment. To err on the side of caution is not a bad thing. I used to fast regularly, sometimes as long as three days. I learned the proper way to ease your body back into a normal rhythm after fasting. Start with liquids, then increase to runny/soft food. Start slow for the best results. No large steaks, greasy soaked fried chicken, greasy burgers, or hard breads. I recall a nurse informing me that medications taken pre- and postsurgery can also mess with the digestive tract and slow it down, which is the next paragraph.

Meds

I was thankful for the meds administered presurgery to put me under or, as I say, "knocked me out." This state of deep sleep is essential and crucial to the success of any surgery. It enables the surgeon to make the necessary incisions and work on the insides without my consciousness getting in his way. The way I see it, the medications paralyze the body and turns the brain off so there is no awareness of any pain (for obvious reasons). Believe me, the pain is still there, your mind is just turned off to it. This is such a precise surgery that the body needs to be in a so-called "frozen state" or, more precisely, in a state of suspended animation. This way, it is much easier for the doc to perform his pinpoint accuracy. I think these specific meds may have played a part in the slow startup of the intestinal tract also. Just a thought of mine here, but you must admire what these surgeons can do for us today. These guys coupled with modern technology and science make a marvelous team. I mean, they go inside a living human body and fix or repair a part of it. To me, it is just a magnificent achievement. I have problems just fixing a simple carburetor on my vintage 1973 Ford pickup truck. Comparing my carburetor work to the surgeons' work would be like me keeping the engine up and running while taking off the intake manifold and replacing it with a new one, and his work has way more sludge accompanied with it, and it's extremely more dangerous.

Postsurgery Tips and Advice

The following few tidbits are for postsurgery care. Some cover the first five days at your house after surgery, some a little longer. The hospital staff will give you a list of do's and don'ts. Please pay attention to their guidelines.

You must listen to this. I am serious here. Limit your activity for the days that you have your catheter in. Listen to me, bro, no thinking like a Neanderthal man at this time. No "I can take it, I'm stronger than anyone else" attitude. Absolutely no running, jumping, hiking, or exercising. Avoid all stairs if possible. If you can't avoid stairs, then at least gradually navigate the stairway, holding tightly to the handrail and at a very slow pace. Better yet, have someone by your side to help you who can aid you. I'm not talking about a little kid at your side holding your hand. I mean someone strong enough to catch you if you begin to stumble. At this point, even a small fall can be very damaging.

Something else you should not be doing. Don't do any heavy lifting. You would be surprised at the amount of pressure you place on the internal organs when lifting anything. It's my personal recommendation that you not lift anything heavier than a half-gallon of milk, and don't even do that for the first two days of postsurgery. I'm saying, "Brother, just try to relax, heal thyself. Even though it is difficult, just try to do nothing." Let someone else help aid you in making your moves, or better yet, stand down and let them do certain things for you. The act of laying around and sleeping most of the day is a good way to heal your body; however, it may be mentally difficult for some people because you may be one of those "always on the go, I'll do it myself" individuals. That's a fine attribute to have when all is healthy, a bad attitude to have during the healing process. It may also be difficult to relax and do nothing because most guys don't want to place the burden on someone else with doing things for them. But believe me, you are going to be in pain and you are on medication, so just give it a try. You want a helper who can understand the seriousness of your situation, maybe even more so than you do and will be glad to assist you. I can't emphasize this enough. "It's great to have someone you can trust standing by your side as you journey down this road." Also important at this time, do not squat down to pick something up. Undue pressure could be placed on the internal areas.

This next one idea is not so obvious, so it needs to be said to you. Don't cross your legs while sitting in a chair because it also can place undue strain on the internal organs, and on all the new incisions, in addition to the areas connected with the Foley catheter. Sit with your legs apart and lean backward; however, when you need to get up, let your partner pull you forward.

Please don't even think about getting behind the steering wheel of a car for two weeks. Remember what was discussed previously—driving can be uncomfortable and dangerous at this time. If, for some reason, you must travel as a passenger by car, don't travel long distances. The bouncing from uneven roads and the stop-and-go flow of normal traffic will be hard on the stitched-up areas, especially those internal stitches. The internal stitches are the ones you can't see but can surely feel as pain. Protect them. No operating large vehicles or machinery. No motorcycle or ATV. *No driving*. This no driving thing should be self-evident, but it bears repeating, especially when you read the attorney's part below. Postsurgery is when you will be taking narcotic medication and should not mix the medications with operating a vehicle. This is not a smart combination. The medication in your system mixed with the pain you will be feeling will make your reaction time slower. Those two reasons, each one by themselves, would slow anyone's reaction time down, but both working together will encourage a third one to arise, and that is having the road work against you, like sharp turns or quick stops. Obviously, you must take care of your health and well-being. You don't want to place yourself in a condition to harm yourself. Worse yet, there are also huge legal ramifications to consider. Let's just hypothesize here for a moment. Suppose you do get behind the wheel and get into an accident. Any attorney worth his salt will find out you are taken medication, and then he'll find out why you are taking medication, and you shouldn't have been operating/driving a motor vehicle due to your medical condition. Say goodbye to your house and maybe a couple years of your life. Don't be stupid.

After eight days or longer, you might feel strong enough to try short drives as a passenger only. I wouldn't consider any cross-country driving for at least two months. This is all for your own good. Take life easy for a few weeks and get your body back to good health, dude, it's only two weeks, you're an adult, you can surely do two weeks. This might help. Remember, you are your strongest weapon against yourself. You have to think about what you are doing. You're the only one who can control what you do. This isn't a sports-related injury where you can stretch your muscles and work your body back into shape quickly.

The only exercises you should be doing while at home and healing are simple leg exercises. For example, let's discuss calf exercises for a moment. Calf exercises are imperative for the prevention of blood clots. Nobody wants a blood clot, and these exercises are easily completed while in a sitting position.

Sit on a chair and stretch out your legs in front of you. With both heels firmly on the ground, lift one of your legs a short distance off the ground, maybe six inches off the ground.

Point your toes out straight as far as you can, which contracts the muscle.

Relax your foot, which will relax the calf muscles.

Now, curl your toes back toward your knee as far as you can. Really curl. This stretches the calf muscle.

Point, relax, curl; so easy and so good for you. Do ten on each leg, one leg at a time. Don't try both legs at the same time. Maybe you can do both legs after you enter into your third week of recovery. Run this one by your doc.

I suggest doing twenty reps on every even hour of the clock. I performed five reps every half hour I was awake. Another exercise, which is equally good for you, is just after you are done with the above calf exercises, try doing this one. While holding only one foot up off the floor, pretend your big toe is a magic marker and try writing the alphabet in midair using all large capital letters.

After completing the above stretches and alphabet writing on the even hours, every odd hour, it would be good to stand up to stretch all the leg muscles. Take a leisurely walk around the inside of your house. The fact is, walking is really good for your leg muscles during this time and helps work your lungs. It's also (believe it or not) great for your digestive tract. It helps in getting the digestive system moving. While walking around, try taking about twenty steps on the tip toes, also great for calf muscles. Stretching your legs like this every hour is beneficial in helping with blood circulation too, which means less chance of a clot forming. Besides, whenever you are standing up or walking around, gravity takes over and helps the drainage of urine while wearing the catheter.

Breathing

Yes, brother, breathing is an exercise. The composition of our human body is amazing, and the way it works is truly astonishing. Our bodies have many strictly voluntary muscles. Just lift you hand up and touch your forehead—that's all voluntary muscles; the hand never lifts itself. However, the human body also has a few involuntary muscles (example, the heart. You never tell it what to do), and we all have some groups of muscles which are both, as in blinking of the eye. When we are asleep, our breathing is completed with involuntary muscles; however, when awake, we can use the very same muscles voluntarily to exercise our lungs by inhaling and exhaling as much air through our lungs as possible, so this becomes a very important exercise, and it should be done correctly and deeply. After any surgery, this breathing exercise becomes significantly important. Postsurgery is often a difficult time to take proper and deep breaths, you're on medication (hint: strong pain meds can slow down your breathing), you're a little drowsy and most of the time laying on your back, so your body just doesn't expend the necessary energy to breathe deeply. This is where our minds come to the rescue. As humans, we must mentally communicate with our physical portion to breathe properly and, even more importantly, breathe *deeply* for the correct air supply to the lungs. Because of this very reason, someone came up with a very cool and special little gadget. This device can actually teach you how to inhale correctly for slow deep breaths, the ones your lungs need to stay healthy. While you're in the hospital, the staff will constantly be checking your blood oxygen level (why? Because the hospital staff knows the importance of proper oxygen levels and deep breathing). Blood oxygen level is how well your lungs distributes oxygen to your cells, and the staff may even administer oxygen to you through a nose tube or a mask to ensure you are breathing correctly and suppling your lungs with the oxygen they need, and really, it's not your lungs that need the oxygen, the lungs are merely a collection device for the oxygen. It's really your red blood cells that *need* the oxygen, and the red blood cells can only get it if your lungs collect it by breathing it in. At home, you will have to do the best you can by yourself. Breathing deeply for multiple reps to get the greatest results. Deep breathing is beneficial for lung function.

The hospital staff is likely to provide you with a special little gadget which I mentioned earlier but only touched on briefly. I'll now talk about it in detail for better understanding of how important this is. It's a rather small device with a rather large name, the "incentive spirometer voldyne 5000." Isn't that a cool name? And if you use your imagination, you can see it as a miniature R2D2 from the original *Star Wars* movie. My own self-described definition of this gadget would be "a small handheld clear plastic, manually-operated, do-it-yourself, lung-motivating breathing unit." The very word *incentive* in its title means motivating and encouragement. I don't know who invented this little device, but trust me, it's brilliant. This little guy helps you inhale the most oxygen you can with each breath you take. Its size is basically six inches square, usually made of clear plastic with two clear vertical cylinders in the middle of the unit— one narrow cylinder, and one wide cylinder. It also has a blue flexible tube protruding straight out toward you from between the two cylinders with a mouth piece at the end of the blue tube. This blue tube and mouth piece is what you "inhale" through. *Do not exhale* into the blue tube, because you will place unneeded moisture inside the unit and mess it up, so always only inhale through the blue tube. As you are holding the device in your right hand and it's facing you, raise it up to eye level and look at the left side narrow cylinder. You will notice that the smaller narrow plastic vertical cylinder has a small yellow puck inside of it, and that puck goes up and down as you inhale. There are a few words printed on the outside of this smaller cylinder and located at its center point. The bottom word is *best*, then *better*, and then *good* at the top. The *good* area is like saying you're slacking off, so go back and try again. This time, keep the small yellow puck floating within the *better* region of the tube. As you get more exercise and your lungs get stronger, shoot for the puck to be held in the *best* region. I'm not sure most people even look at this left-hand narrow cylinder or the words printed on it. I know I didn't at first. I looked at the wider/larger cylinder located on the right side of the blue intake tube. This cylinder also has a puck in it, usually white. This larger cylinder is where most of the action takes place, and consequently, this action really draws your attention. The wider cylinder measures the volume of air that you inhale or, in physician's terms, the "ml's volume of intake."

Now, to operate this device, hold it in front of you at eye level with your right hand, and with your left hand, hold the blue flex tube. Before you place the blue flex tube to your mouth, exhale as much air as you can. I mean really exhale. Exhale into the ambient air around you and not into the device. Force yourself to exhale as never before so you can inhale like never before. Deeper exhalations are important; obviously, the greater volume you exhale, the greater the volume of air you can inhale. Inhaling will raise the white measuring disc which is inside the wider/larger right-hand side cylinder (this measuring disc looks like a small white hockey puck). The higher the white hockey puck goes, the greater volume of air is taken into your lungs, and naturally, the better the results you'll have. You want the right-hand side white puck to go as high as you can make it go while keeping the left side yellow puck in the region of *better*. It may be difficult on your first couple of tries, but first tries are just that—a try.

My father would tell me, "Nothing starts at the top unless you're digging a hole." As you continue with multiple attempts at using this device, you will notice that it gets easier to inhale more air as you try to exhale more air; your alveoli are working. Believe me, you will get better with each succeeding try. Better exhaling is the secret to better inhaling. The optimum level of success while using this device is to have the small left-hand yellow puck be held up in the *best* region and the right-hand white puck in the 2,500 or more region. Keep on trying, I'm confident that you will use it correctly. If you don't make it to the 2,500, do your best and record the results. Next time, beat your last time results.

Our human lungs are tremendously specialized structures and should be considered very precious by everyone because they are essential for life. Our wonderful lungs breathe in new air and exhale out the old air the body doesn't need and can't use. Here's a Budd note: When I'm using the word *air*, it's just a general term for the stuff we breathe in and truly need, but the amazing thing about our wonderful air is we can't see any of it. Each of the approximately 20,000 breaths of air we humans breath in and out daily is comprised of numerous components. The largest component of the air is nitrogen (approximately 78 percent), followed by oxygen (approximately 20 percent), and about 1 percent water (moisture), then many other trace components like argon gas, carbon dioxide, and even some methane. However, our specialized lungs are searching only for that one enchanted component we all love and is known as oxygen.

Oxygen is the main component our blood cells and brain need, and that's what the lungs are reaching for. The lungs take in oxygenated air and almost magically de-oxygenate it, keeping the oxygen inside the body and exhaling all the excess components that are not needed. You have to admit, our lungs are highly praised and sophisticated pieces of equipment, and I, for one, am thankful we have them to help us. Your lungs do this miraculous exchanging trick by using tiny little balloon-like sacs called *alveoli* (al-vee-oh-ly). These little sacs look like microscopic bunches of grapes, and they are very, very, very, very tiny. In fact, your body has about three hundred million alveoli for each lung! That's an astronomically large number! An astounding grand total of six hundred million small bunches of grapes inside both our lungs! Which means they must be extremely tiny. As we inhale, we take into our lung's good oxygen, and the little alveoli grapes gobbles it up like a bunch of little Pac-men and sends it into your blood stream to all our vital organs. Once used up, the blood stream brings back all the waste products (carbon dioxide) our body makes, and again, the alveoli exchange it, and the lungs exhale it all out. All that in order to breath in more oxygen, which completes the cycle. Again, the more you exhale, the more you can you inhale. Think about that the next time you breathe in and out. Six hundred million tiny alveoli are hard at work keeping you healthy, and you didn't even know it. However, here's the kicker; you must breathe deep to keep all six hundred million working. If you don't take those deep breaths, then some of the alveoli are not working. If all alveoli are not working, then some get a little sad, so please, for your own good, take those deep, deep breaths and make them all happy again.

I recommend taking six complete cycles of deep breaths during your lung exercise while using the spirometer 5000 machine. Now, once you have this deep breathing exercise down and understand what they do for you, you can also deep breath anytime during the day without the spirometer machine. The machine is to keep you toeing the line and doing the breathing exercises correctly and completely. We all have a tendency to shorten things, like only doing nine pushups instead of ten and thinking, *That's good enough, I'll do ten tomorrow*. Yeah, right.

Something else for your enlightenment. While you are standing there using the spirometer machine, after a few large exhales and the adjoining big inhales, you might experience a slight feeling of dizziness. If you are of a certain age, you might say, "Wow, dude, like, I just got a head rush." This rush may come after about the fourth or fifth cycle of deep breathing. There is no need to worry about this dizziness. In fact, you want that woozy feeling. You should strive for that head rush feeling. What you are really experiencing is a rush of fresh new oxygen-rich blood flowing into your brain because your lungs are working at full speed, and that, my friend, is good for you. If you don't feel a little dizzy after your fourth cycle, then you might not be doing it correctly, perhaps not exhaling fully enough. Try again. Here's another key note. You need to go to the extreme at both ends. The more air you exhale, the larger volume of new air you'll be able to inhale. The more you inhale, the higher the white puck will rise, and consequently, the more you will be able to exhale, and the cycle continues. The higher the puck rises, the more you exercise those little alveoli, and the stronger they will become. Exercising them is how you strengthen them. It is a marvelous cycle, but you have to make it work. The more you exercise your body, the stronger your body will become. It's the same with your lungs too. As your lungs become stronger, the more oxygen you can take in, and of course, the more oxygen you take in, the better you feel and the healthier you become. I still have my incentive spirometer, and I keep it on top of my refrigerator. I use it a couple of times a week. I learned from the nurse while I was in the hospital that it is important to breathe correctly. She took the time to instruct me on the proper use of spirometer and the alveoli we have in our lungs.

One interesting fact about the spirometer is the adjustable marker attached to the outside of the large clear cylinder on the right. It's usually yellow in color, and it slides up and down, which allows you to place the marker in the position where the white puck rises up on your first inhale. This first mark is the one you try to beat each time you do these breathing exercises. With each additional exhale and then inhale cycle, you should be able to draw in slightly more air than the previous cycle so you can try to beat your last mark. Back in the late '60s and '70s, people were practicing this method of deep inhaling and didn't even know it.

Each day, while practicing your breathing exercises on your third or fourth breath, you should be able to inhale enough air to raise the white puck inside the larger cylinder higher than the yellow adjustable marker on the outside. You can then raise the yellow marker to your new higher point. The trick is when you use the spirometer, on your second or third breath, you need to try to match the yellow marker's level or, better yet, try to beat that level and go somewhat higher. Obviously, there is a point where you will peak out, but that peak is what you want to strive for. This way, you know you are utilizing all the happy alveolis in your lungs and that your lungs are getting a good work out.

Each new day, when you do you first inhale, you'll find the white puck might not raise up to your last level of the yellow marker. Keep in mind that's OK. Failing on your first attempt is no big deal. The big deal is for you to keep on trying because on your second attempt, you might get closer to the mark, and on your third try, you might just meet it or surpass it. Look at Thomas Edison. The man failed thousands of times, but he kept right on trying. In fact, he once said, "I have now learned a thousand ways it won't work." Besides, you should look at the word *fail* differently; actually, it's really an acronym for "First Attempt In Learning."

That sounds great; however, I want to go a bit further and say, "Well-managed failure can lead to success."

Urine Monitoring

While at home recovering, there will be uncertain times full of trials and tribulations. You will surely be tired and probably feel drowsy most of the time and likely have strange pains from the surgery, several incisions to keep clean and protect from damage, and medication to take on a timely schedule. You have to exercise your legs frequently and deep sleep you surely long for but can't seem to get, checking the urine flow, and other normal things you have to do for your condition. That's all OK and fades away a little with each passing day, so just bear through it. Tough times don't last, tough people do. Your new friend, Mr. Foley D. Catheter, takes care of the urine problem and is something you must contend with along with all of its encumbrance. I'll just throw this idea out one more time, and although it might be hard to accomplish, nonetheless, if you could, try to close up your life a little and retreat inside your house. It would be a good idea, during this time, to collect your thoughts and embrace these changes. It will do you a world of good. Like all gentleman in the first week postsurgery, I needed to wake up every couple of hours to take the medicines at their prescribed times (which was every couple hours) and make sure the catheter wasn't tangled on something and it was draining correctly and monitor my urine output. I also needed to get up frequently to stretch my legs. Many times, you might wake up just because you may have that full bladder feeling, which is completely normal. Your schedule is just messed up temporarily. This waking up frequently was a two-edged sword. I didn't like it, but it did feel good to walk around and stretch my legs, especially my calves. The flowing of urine is important, and you need to monitor the amount coming out. If it's not coming out on a regular basis or if it is not fairly clear in color, you may have a problem; however, you won't know if you don't monitor. In order to have more fluids coming out, you need to have more going in, and with the medications you are consuming, it is a very good idea to push the liquids a lot. More liquids help in the circulation those meds. While wearing the catheter, plenty of liquids is a good thing. When the liquids come out, they carry bodily waste products out, which helps in keeping you healthy. Plus, while the catheter is in, you can drink as much liquids as you can handle because they pass right through your system. No time to stop and get stale in the bladder. They travel along their merry way, so drink, drink, drink.

If you are consuming an adequate amount of liquids, your body will be continuously producing urine every second of every day; it literally never stops (more involuntary muscles at work). The liquid you are producing ends up in your body's holding tank (bladder). Remember, your surgeon had to cut and reconnect the urethra pipeline, so monitoring the outflow of urine is an important indication of the success of your operation. If done successfully, the flow of urine will be painless, and you will have a continual flow into the collection bag. If it is not coming out seamlessly and painlessly, there may be a problem inside. Also monitor the color of urine. If you are experiencing unusual or increasing pain in your waist area or are seeing more than just a few spots of blood in the catheter or no urine flow at all, call your doc. My urine flow was painless and continually dripping down the tube, so monitoring my flow indicated a successful operation and helped in easing my thoughts. For the entire twelve days, I only saw a few small red solid globs of blood, which were minor blood clots, and the clots did not come out all at once; they were spread out over time. My clots were few and bright red in color. They only appeared for the first couple of days and then cleared out altogether. Another indication of success.

Here's a thought. Where does all the outflow come from? Obviously, it comes from the fluids you take in, so I recommend you monitor the amount of fluids you're taking in as well, and you might do good by writing this intake information down. I visually monitored and physically recorded all of the in/out fluid activities daily using a pencil and paper log sheet. Here's something cool. I recorded all the different amounts using a unit of measurement called milliliters rather than ounces just for the fun of it. My decision to use milliliters was based on the language doctors and hospitals use. They all communicated using dosages of medicine measured in milliliters, and I thought it would be fun to talk to them in their own language. My father introduced me to the usefulness of numbers at a young age, and as the years passed, I turned into a bit of a mathematician. Since I grew up with an extensive use of mathematics in the science of reading and understanding blueprints for the buildings we worked on in the family business. Now after studying the doctor's language of milliliters, I began to understand how easy this system of numbers was to use and to calculate, I found it to be a far better measurement system than our present-day system of using ounces, cups, quarts, and gallons.

I'm still an all-American, red-blooded male, so no letters of condemnation about quarts and gallons please; besides, everything is already measured in the metric system. You just have to look. It's there. For example, when I was young, all the car engines were measured in cubic inches (CI's) the famous 327 CI's engine and the big block 454 CI engine. Now, there's not an auto maker on the planet that uses CI's, all engines are metrically measured as three-liter, four-liter, five-liter, and so on. Even soda pop comes in a two-liter bottle. I've noticed a few one-liter bottles of water on the convenient store shelves. Almost every kitchen measuring cup has both U.S. ounces and millimeters printed on the side. Look at the everyday soda can in your house. Twelve fl. oz. right. Look closer. See the 355 mL both printed in plain sight. You can't find any liquid-filled container that doesn't list both U.S. and metric on the same label. Even the pickle jar has them. Check out the bag of bread we all purchase weekly at the store. That's right, it has both. Take a good look at the labels of any food which has the "nutrition facts" printed on the label, all the cholesterol, saturated fat, sodium, calcium, and the host of other items, they all are measured in milligrams, and if larger, they use grams. The metric system, brother, is already here. You're the one that has to change now. The metric system is founded on a unit measurement of 1000. That number is easy to divide into smaller parts or easy to go larger too. 1000 mL's equal 1 liter, 2000 mL's equal 2 liters, which is the size of the 2-liter bottle of soda at the grocery store. However, that's adding up in volume. When you go down in volume, it goes like this. 236 mL's equal 1 fluid cup, going down further, 29 mL's equals 1 fluid oz. Now this is where the problem becomes apparent. One ounce is about as small as U.S. scale efficiently goes, but you can see the mL's still has twenty-nine more increments to go smaller with. Nevertheless, as we as humans need to go smaller than an ounce, much smaller, the metric system is great at going smaller. As we approach the smaller end of the U.S. measuring scale, it gets difficult to divide ounces into smaller and smaller parts but very easy to divide millimeters. You begin to see why it is easier and more efficient to measure out doses of medications in mL's instead of ounces. It's relatively easy to keep going smaller and smaller in milliliters. This is where the metric system wins, when a pharmacist or doctor has to measure out a precise amount of medicine, especially within a syringe, which must be done correctly and with outstanding precision. The metric classifications makes calculating very small volumes convenient. The use of millimeters let you dial into a highly precise measured amount, extremely more precise than our present-day measurement of ounces could ever do. There's no comparison—the metric system wins hands down.

Well, once again, I have gotten off track. Monitor your fluids on a daily basis and record the info. By recording the outflow and intake of fluids, you'll know each day how much your intake really is and, consequentially, how much outflow is. After my surgery, while at home recovering, I tried for a daily minimum intake of approximately 1,900 milliliters of liquid, which equals approx. 64 ounces, and that amount, I believe, is the FDA recommended daily intake for Americans. Most of the time, I ran over and approached 90 ounces a day. On the down side, I noticed that both the daily intake and outflow never did match up with each other. After some research, I discovered this is normal since, some days, you may take in more fluid than you can easily measure. For instance, if you had a bowl of chicken noodle soup for lunch, it's difficult to measure precisely the amount of liquid in the bowl, so it becomes a guesstimate. Perhaps on a hot day, you will sweat more than the next, then you may have less outflow than intake. The numbers will never precisely match, but this gives you a good estimated figure. The reason monitoring is valuable is you don't want to see a much larger intake than outflow, especially during the first few days postsurgery. If you experience a larger number of intake fluids, a small outflow, and increasing pain, call the doc. It will indicate a problem.

Since your body produces urine outflow on a constant twenty-four hours a day, drip-by-drip basis, you will notice that every time you stand up, some fluid will flow down the catheter tubing. After sitting for a while, I would stand up and see about 45 mL's coming down the tube (45 is equal to 1.5 ounces). Additionally, after a long nap I would look at the measurement lines printed on the measuring bag and notice the fluid would sometimes amount to approximately 150 mL's (5 ounces).

The mornings after I was finally able to get some much-needed sleep, perhaps five solid hours, which was about the seventh day post-surgery, I awoke with a tremendous urge to urinate. You may also experience this as well, which is understandable while wearing the catheter. It doesn't take a lot of fluid accumulation in the bladder to produce this urge to urinate. Again, it's partly due to the funnel shaped balloon device pressing against the bladders wall. Anyway, I got out of bed, stood up straight, and watched the fluid flow down the tube and into the measuring bag. It's quite incredible to watch the draining of fluids without my brain issuing any directions. My body was doing quite well on its own with no help from me. The total which came out that morning was approximately 200 mL's (around 6.5 ounces, the most so far). Occasionally, I noticed the color of the urine would change. I'm guessing the color would be determined by what I drank hours before.

As I stated, I tried to drink a lot of fluids—about ten ounces every hour for the first seven hours of my day. As long as I continued consuming that amount of fluids (the majority of fluid was water), the urine was basically clear. Ten ounces of fluids every hour may seem like a lot to drink for most people, but on the contrary, it's quite healthy for you and is easy to accomplish if you approach it in a systematic way. I used the simple and handy Dixie five-ounce paper cup. They're always available, always clean, and easy to use. I'd fill the little cup up with whatever fluid I desired and just down it quickly. Downing this small amount—five ounces—of water or juice once every thirty minutes is not difficult to accomplish, and of course, five ounces every half hour is ten ounces every hour—easy. The small Dixie cup makes it convenient. When you have a variety of medications to take throughout the day, these small cups are not only convenient but make it easy to take the medication as well as achieving the goal of measuring your fluid intake. (Take one pill and use one full Dixie cup, five ounces, easy as pie.)

In fact, I made a game out of drinking this amount of fluid. In reality, trying to consume a large glass filed with eight ounces of any liquid and doing it once every hour and doing it multiple times (eight times) per day every day can get somewhat tiring and tedious too.

This is where the little Dixie cup becomes a star and is the smarter way to go since they were so manageable. The game I played was to start my day with two Dixie cups of fresh water (ten ounces) before anything else. After that, as the day went on, the next five ounces of fluids would be orange juice, then thirty minutes later, it would be another type of juice (cranberry, grape, or my all-time favorite—POM, the classic red pomegranate juice). I would change it up and go in a different direction like filling the Dixie cup half full of water and the other half with orange juice, just mixing various juice concoctions like half-pomegranate and half-cranberry—easy and convenient. I even made some raisin juice. Hot boiling water, big handful of raisins, then puréed in the blender. Plus, a five-ounce Dixie cup is easier. It's not like the eight-ounce glass every hour. That's arduous. If you nap through an hour or two, it's pretty easy to catch up using these little cups.

About a month or so before my surgery, while doing our grocery shopping, I discovered these cool little cherry fruit cups manufactured by the Del Monte Company. Wow, did these guys come in handy while I was at home recuperating. They come ready-made in convenient four-ounce cups. I discovered that with my Ninja blender, I could place four of these Del Monte ready-made cups of cherry fruit cocktail into the blender and then add four full Dixie cups of water (thus adding more water to my intake) and literally turned this water and fruit mixture into a universal and smooth liquid fruit drink. Add some ice, and you can blend it all together and you have a really good homemade fruit smoothie. I poured it into a glass decanter and kept that refrigerated. It was easy to have that mixture ready in the refrigerator for me to take out and pour into the little five-ounce Dixie cups and down it with tasty comfort every half hour and also if I was supposed to take my medications. It was so very tasty, it actually made me want to drink more which, in turn, helped me achieve my fluid intake goals. You can't see me right now, but I'm patting myself on my back for that idea.

Later on in your recovery, you can start to introduce a wider variety of liquids into your diet like coffee, tea, more types of juice, soda pop, and if you're taking different types of vitamins, the color of your urine will likely change. One morning, I grabbed the Ninja blender and made myself some fresh orange juice with a slight difference. I peeled four oranges, cut up two bananas, added ten ounces of cold water, a few ice cubes, and liquefied it. Sweet. It was so tasty, I drank all of it within ninety minutes. Wow overload. Way too fast with an extra bonus of a couple of brain freezes along the way. Later on, like several hours later, I noticed the color of my urine wasn't as clear as before. I don't know for sure. I'm guessing that perhaps a little of the pulp from the oranges or their color were showing up in my urine.

I didn't drink any coffee, alcohol, or soda (which I don't drink much of anyway) for two weeks before surgery, and I didn't drink any of those the entire time I had the catheter (twelve days). I also didn't have any for two months thereafter. I drank mostly fruit juices by themselves or mixed with water. I also drank a lot of milk—love that milk—and now I found a new drink. It's called "Vanilla Soymilk," and I'm hooked on it. I use it in my cereal, in my tea, and at least two or three Dixie cups of just straight soymilk per day. I drank a lot of fluids while I was recovering. Even today, I strive for at least 1750 milliliters per day. It isn't uncommon for me (because I drink a lot) to go up to 2900 mL's per day (roughly 98 ounces). I must tell ya, after the catheter is removed, don't even hit the 50 ounces a day mark. Anything above 50 will be too much.

The different fruit juices I made while wearing the catheter were: white grape juice, homemade blueberry juice (very tasty), orange juice with pulp (gotta have pulp), apple and cranberry juice(good for the GI tract), Gatorade, POM, and even a half-quart of black currant juice, tart and sweetened cherry juice, tomato juice (tomato juice is good over ice on a hot day or hot out of the microwave on a cold day). I even found berry-flavored Aloe Vera juice at a whole foods store, and lastly, good old-fashioned prune juice. I'm sure you're thinking, prune juice, *yuck*, who voluntarily does that! I'm one of the few weird guys on the planet who likes the taste of prune juice. It goes way back to my childhood days when I suffered a kinked colon (which I mentioned earlier). I also noticed a change of color in the urine because of the various fluids I consumed. I also continued to keep a daily log measuring the amount of urine I emptied from the measuring bag and the time of day I emptied it. Strange, it always seemed as though I took in a little more than what came out. Not a large or concerning difference.

My measuring bag that was strapped to my leg for twelve days, when full, held 400 mL's (1.7 cups or approx. 14 ounces). I waited until it was filled up to the 400 mL's mark before emptying it. It was easier for me to record the amounts and compare them on the chart when I kept the number always at 400. It is such an even number and helped with my recordkeeping. I'll relay a thought to you here, and that is, in retrospect, if I had to go through this again, I might not wait until reaching the full 400 mL's. I would probably change to every 300 mL's (10 fluid oz.) or even the 200 mark. That 200 mark would be easier to handle, and if you are going to measure yours and record it, you might want to do the same. The few days that I actually did my precise measuring, I had to be extra cautious because of the fullness of that measuring bag strapped to my leg. At 400, it would be quite heavy and extremely awkward walking at times (had to walk slow), especially when it was beginning to reach the full mark. Just think for a moment about taping a full can of Coca Cola to your ankle and walking around your house with it all day. 200 mL's would be much more convenient. The times of day I emptied the measuring bag varied depending on the volume of intake or, in other words, rate of consumption, but that seems reasonable. I would sometimes force myself to drink more liquids than normal and check my chart just for fun. During the times I consumed more fluids, I obviously filled the 400 mL measuring bag more quickly.

A friend of mine who knew what I was going through brought over a large bowl of freshly cut-up fruit—cantaloupe, pears, strawberries, blueberries, honeydew melon, and a bowl of my all-time favorite watermelon. I was in fruit heaven for a few days. I enjoy eating fruit more than anything else, and I find them to be quite healthy. I must say, I get a little sugar rush when I indulge too much on the fruit. However, if you have a task that you must get done, grab a watermelon and eat five or six big slices, and you'll see what I mean. Is it a sugar rush or just a plain old-fashioned energy boost?

Maybe it doesn't matter, fruit is just tasty to eat. Don't get me wrong, I'm still a good old Colorado boy and enjoy a fine cut of barbecue or healthy burger hot off the grill, but fruit will always be the king. Plus, unlike meat, fruits come in their own convenient air-tight containers and are ready to eat anywhere you take it and at any time. Try doing that with a cheeseburger. I noticed that while I was drinking my usual amount of fluids and consuming all this luscious fruit, I was pumping out the fluids in double time! Seriously, it seemed like every thirty-five or forty minutes, that full bladder urge would begin to ring in my head, and I would have to stand up and drain the fluids.

For me, it was a hard time for the first few days after arriving home from the hospital. I could only nap for two hours at any one time, had pain most of the time, plus I had medications to take at specific but different times (like every two to three hours), and for this, I used my handy Dixie cups. After taking whatever meds were scheduled for me at the time, I would clean up a little (wash face/brush teeth) and then gently stretch my arms, do a few breathing exercises, and prepare for several walking laps around the inside of my house to work my legs and calf muscles and drain some fluids. This all tired me out so much that I would return to the bedroom or my recliner and nap 'til the alarm rang for the next round of pills. Thank God for that recliner! It quickly became my favorite piece of furniture. I used it so much, my wife suggested I just Velcro it to my back! She's so funny sometimes! Here's my advice. If you don't have a reclining chair, borrow one. You'll need it for a good month. It's quite comfortable, and the extra benefit is they're adjustable, so if you get tired of one position, you can change your position for extended comfort. Use it in the sitting-up position, laying-down position, or a host of in between. Besides the recliner, an extra good thing is a soft and comfortable floor-length robe, because it will be the easiest piece of clothing to wear. It's too difficult to get fully dressed for many reasons. Main reason being you have the catheter attached to you, but also, you are in mild discomfort because of the operation and you can't move fast. It is also difficult to bend over, so trying to get dressed is just out of the question. So you might as well just be comfortable. For those four days, I wore nothing but my catheter and floor-length robe. I never did that before. You're not going to be able to wear a pair of pants at this time, so a floor-length robe and, later on, an oversized pair of sweat pants are good. If you don't have a robe or sweats, get them before the operation date.

OK, back to measuring the liquids. The following chart is a measurement table that I maintained on my fluids. At the time, I was charting this information, and because of my mathematical interest, I tried to keep everything standard and only emptied the holding bag when it reached up to the 400 ml mark. A little difficult to accomplish, so I hope you enjoy the chart. I crunched numbers every day and wanted to see what was happening. It was a good way to be more in tune with my body's recovery process as well as passing some time while I was at home recuperating. I'm glad I kept this information, because now I can pass it on to you. This is just one of many daily charts I maintained. This particular measurement chart shows the highest outflow of liquids.

Chart of mL's Outflow—Twenty-four hours

1:16 a.m.	400 mL's
5:11 a.m.	400 mL
9:34 a.m.	400 mL
Noon	400 mL
3:41 p.m.	400 mL
8:00 p.m.	400 mL
1:00 a.m.	400 mL

The chart above and its 24-hour period is from 1:16 a.m. until 1:00 a.m. the next morning. Adding up all the 400 MLs x 7 emptying's of the collection bag = 2,800 milliliters (94 ounces). As long as the catheter is in place, you can drink an ocean of water and it won't matter. Now, the normal everyday urine range for a human body to put out is about 1850 ml's or about 62 ounces, and that is supposed to be average, and 68 ounces is quite easy for us humans to intake in

24 hours, so my readings are right on target but being just above the normal; however, I really do strive to take in a lot of fluids each day. Remember, urine is waste product. The level of 400 ml's always had to be the constant element in this equation, but obviously, the length of time between changes varied. The time varied because I had to wait for the fluid level to reach 400 before draining. You can also see the different times of day, which is why I mentioned getting yourself ready for a strange sleep/wake cycle. You might be in the middle of a nap and the alarm will go off, notifying you it's time to take another one of the many meds you'll be on.

Oh yes, I'm glad I mentioned "the alarm." Budd note alert: I might as well inform you right here, it's a good idea to set your cell phone alarm to alert you for the different times you must take your medications. There are different meds you have to take, and you take them at different times. One medication I took every four hours, one med was every six hours, and the pain meds were every three hours or when needed. So when you first start to take your meds, all is fine and dandy, but as time goes on, the time you have to take those meds gets mixed up and confusing pretty fast. An alarm is a helping hand at this time because you may be napping when it's time to take another pill, and you shouldn't miss a time. Another super good idea is to get a large sheet of white poster board and draw a gird system on it, lay it down flat on your kitchen countertop, Scotch Tape it down so it can't be move around, and set each bottle of meds at the top of each grid and label each square going down the page with the time of day and date for each one of the medications. You have to add the date as you go down the page on the grid because you will be taking meds for multiple days. This grid system worked great and kept me from messing up the pills and their taking times. This way, I wouldn't take a pill I wasn't supposed to take or taking a pill at the wrong time, because it can be confusing, so the chart is a helping hand. Once you have taken the med, you simply use a sharpie to cross off the square containing the dosage you took and time of day you took it and then set the alarm for the taking of the next pill. The taking times are so spread out over the twenty-four-hour day, and because you will be sleeping or napping a lot, you will tend to get confused quite quickly.

I had to use an alarm and my grid system or I would have missed some of the times I was supposed to take my meds. Wrong meds at the wrong times are not good my friend.

Anyway, back to all the fluids. While at one of my presurgery doctor office consultations, one doc was asking me numerous questions, and the topic of healthy fluid intake came up. Well, as you can tell by now, I'm proud of my fluid consumption which is at least 64 ounces a day and up to 100 on hot summer days, the more you consume, the more hydrated you are, and the more poisons are washed out of your body. As I was proudly describing to him all the wonderful different concoctions of juices and bragging about my 64 ounces or more of fluid intake daily, suddenly, his eye brows went up, leaded toward me, and very quickly jumped into my sentence and stated, "Once the catheter is removed, Budd, you should not consume that much liquid on a daily basis. No one should. It will be too much." He didn't elaborate on that statement, although he did say there are some issues that can arise with too much fluid. He quickly advised me to cut the amount in half. "50 ounces would be advisable, and spread that over an entire 24-hour day." I was proud of my intake, but when that was said, he cut me to the quick, and I just went silent. In hindsight, I wish I would have gone further and inquired of him why he thought I should cut the liquids by half. He didn't clarify his statement, and I didn't ask either. *Bam*, a mistake was just made, and I was going to pay for it later. He quickly went on to other more important instructions for me during my pre and postsurgery issues.

Me not inquiring more on the reduced fluids and him not elaborating on the fluid issue caused me one more rollercoaster ride in my feelings of uncertainty on this journey. However, unknowingly, I was going to find out on my own what the good doc meant about the amount of fluids being cut in half. Man, did I ever find out. You see, while our friendly little buddy, the catheter, is in place, it didn't matter how many fluid ounces I ingested; the more, the merrier. I could have gone over 100 ounces every day because the catheter and bag did everything for me that I would normally do on my own. The catheter took control over the flow of urine. Starting at the bladder, through the tube, and out to the external bag, the flow was completely controlled twenty-four-hours a day, not by me, but by the catheter's system. It's sort of like being an infant baby, you just drain yourself whenever its time. All you do is stand up. The whole process is in an autopilot controlled state. Here's the problem in a nut shell: When the catheter system is removed, the cool autopilot control system is removed as well. The catheter again is a wonderful device and performs its functions quite well, and it did all the work for my body, so I was able to concentrate on healing myself. After the healing process is further along and the catheter is no longer needed, the catheter is obviously removed and *bam*, you have very little control, nothing like you had before surgery. It's like being in a different world. After the catheter removal, you must gradually begin to exercise the sphincter muscles at the bladder area in order for those muscles to gain strength to withstand the force of gravity trying to pull urine out of your body and also just the simple pressure buildup from all the accumulating fluids within the bladder. The pressure buildup will push out some fluids by itself, gravity will pull out some fluids by itself; however, both of those forces working together will defeat your powers easily. So until you are able build up the strength of your own sphincters muscles and be able to overthrow the evil empire and the dreaded drips, cut the fluids down to fifty a day. You must—you'll have no choice. Listen to me. I'm telling you straight up.

I read some informational brochures on this subject and was informed by one doctor that, once the catheter was removed, I would not have the bladder control I had presurgery, but nowhere in all the literature did I read that you have "zero control." I read a lot of information and talked to many people who had also gone through this surgery, and again, no one ever mentioned the word "zero" to me. I truly believed, from all the info, that I knew what was to come and what I should expect. I expected to have some control, and I was prepared for *some* control. I wasn't prepared for *zero* control. However, I'm smart enough to know that any result would be far better than my good friend Paul's outcome was. Now comes the part where I find out why the doc said to me, "Cut the fluids in half." It wasn't until my Foley catheter was removed that I really began to understand my situation and why the doc instructed me to cut my daily intake of fluids in half. I was doing myself an injustice by not cutting down on the amount of fluids. I also felt that I was not provided with the proper instructions of this part of the process. Everyone just sort of touched lightly or breezed over this little detail. To me, this was a big detail to miss. Again, doctors are busy, I can't expect them to detail every detail. So once again, I'm passing a morsel of information onto you so you won't be caught off guard, and I'm hoping your lack of control won't be as bad as what I experienced. It's really just a matter of simple physics. It's not that the surgery was a botched job; the problem was me. I was filling up my bladder with far more fluids than I had the muscle power to control another rollercoaster ride.

The very afternoon the catheter was removed, I experienced the full effect of incontinence, and of course, I was thinking, *Oh my God, what did I just do to myself? Is this going to be my life now? Is this my future?* I mean, I got to tell you guys, this was a far cry from the drips of urine some of the pamphlets, brochures, and books discussed.

Nobody said, "Listen, dude, you may not be able to turn off the kitchen faucet. It's going to run." Drips, I could handle; little, squirts I could handle; but the amount coming out was beyond what I was told about, beyond what I read about, and beyond the expected. To say the least, it was rather disturbing, and I was totally upset about my wet underwear. Think of it this way—take a two-liter bottle of soda, hold it upside down, unscrew the cap 'til it comes off. Now, while still holding it upside down and soda is coming out, try to replace the cap. Now you got the idea. I was thinking the absolute worst for my future. More on this in the next chapter.

Space for notes:

CHAPTER 7

Incontinence

Incontinence and Other Fun Side Effects

Incontinence is an issue of uncontrollable drips (or squirts) of urine, and simply put, it's the result of a weak sphincter or perhaps damaged nerves which run through this area which all leads to lack of control over urination. Your sphincter muscle is a circular muscle which controls the flow of urine out of the bladder and is located just below the base of the bladder. The whole thing is like your kitchen sink faucet. As the water is coming out, you easily turn the handle, and the flow of water slows down until it stops. Easy. You do this every day. The sphincter circular muscles will slowly squeeze the urethra. Same force as the kitchen handle, the urine slows downs 'til it stops.

At this point in my journey, I'm dealing day by day with very slight bladder incontinence. It's very minor now compared to the severity it was at first, like I was explaining in the last chapter. With the catheter in, my sphincter wasn't controlling anything, it was just laying back and enjoying a free ride. Today, the drips only happen to me when there is some stress placed on the bladder e.g., lifting something heavy, sneezing, or running. It's not a full stream of urine, only some little droplets, but it does happen and can be a bummer. It's a small hassle that I don't like and really wish I didn't have, but this is my new normal, and I'm dealing with it. This next sentence is a little embarrassing, but if I force a fart, a few drops come out. Funny, huh? Yeah, go ahead and have a good laugh. I mentioned earlier that I wasn't going to sugarcoat anything, and I want to be honest in my description of my journey. After doing some studying on my own concerning this matter, I found that many professionals have assigned four different categories to incontinence. The four are as follows—stress, urge, overflow, and total. Thank the good lord above I don't have total lack of control. I know what that's like. I experienced it for about a week because, after the catheter was removed, it was total lack of control, and now, I am getting control back, which is great. It took some time and it took work and dedication to control it with lots of Kegel exercising and will possibly be with me the rest of my life. But then again, like my wife stated many times to me, "I'm glad you are here, Budd, and we can deal with it."

As I stated in the last chapter, after my catheter was removed, urine was coming out and I had cero control. For months, I leaked all the time. It happened while I was sitting down or trying to stand up, going upstairs, going downstairs, bending over to pick something up, pulling the grocery cart out of the stack of carts at the grocery store, walking around inside the store, and doing just about anything at any time and, unfortunately, anywhere. In other words, the kitchen faucet was stuck in the open position. After surgery, the first entire week was a wreck and the next week was no better. Well, maybe a little better, but only a tiny bit. Maybe my situation was a little different because I had the catheter in twice the length of time as normal. Like we discussed, the normal length of time to wear the catheter is about six or seven days. Perhaps my muscles atrophied a bit more than they normally would have, or perhaps there was a bit of nerve damage during the operation, and at the very start, I was still pushing the large fluid intake. At this time, about five years after my surgery, I'm back up to at least sixty-four ounces a day, and many times, especially in the warm months, I may shoot up to ninety-plus ounces a day. I'm a firm believer in lots of fluids for better health. My grandfather told me long time ago, "It's how the body rids the impurities." I know if I would slow down on my daily intake, I would experience a slowdown of the droplets coming out. In my life, there will, unfortunately, always be some, and with my high intake, I probably have more than normal.

Anyway, two days after the catheter removal, I did indeed slow down and reduce the amount of my fluid intake. I did what the good doc suggested and cut the amount in half. It was obvious I had to cut it in half—I had no choice. I was running out of clean underwear fast! Even after a couple of weeks, I had very little control over the dripping of urine. Sometimes it wasn't just the little drips, it was the little squirts of urine that happened at random terrible situations. That's right, I said, "Squirts." I'll wait for you to stop smirking. I'm not going to sugarcoat the truth. You need to hear it, especially if you are going through it too. It was terrible. It was dreadful. I mean, just sitting down or bending over to tie my shoes, coughing, sneezing, or simply picking up a gallon of milk, and *bam!* Out comes a little squirt. It can be embarrassing, and I can honestly say it was an emotional letdown. However, here's some good news: Medical advances happen every day, and the surgeons are getting better at the nerve sparing operations, so hopefully, this may not be a large problem to you.

It's really hard to be a badass when you are standing there and you feel that you have just peed your pants. It changed my whole attitude. After the third day post removal, I started to wear man diapers, which helped my underwear situation, thank god for them. They now caught all the drips, and I would have continued to wear them if the situation hadn't started to improve. However, my situation did improve, and about the third week, I could see a very small improvement, but it took exercise. Like I said, I drastically cut down on the fluids which helped in my situation and began the specialized exercises my good doc Jeffery instructed me to do. Both of these used in combination caused a noticeable improvement. Of course, my situation was so dreadful in the beginning that even a little improvement would have been noticeable and welcomed. I'm thankful for the man diapers; they worked great at catching everything. Amen to them. Listen, even if nobody tells you about this little development or if the doc doesn't elaborate the reasons why you should limit your fluid intake, take this advice from me: Until you get those muscles strengthened, cut down on all fluids. In fact, write this down because it is a bit of upright advice. Two days before your scheduled catheter removal, begin to reduce your fluid intake. Drop down to fifty ounces like the doc said. You'll be doing yourself a huge favor.

The good doc Jeffery instructed me on the proper technique for these specialized exercises to help me and even took some time to guide me through several reps of them while in his office to ensure I was doing them correctly—very considerate of him. Believe me, you can do them wrong, and if so, you will not get the best results, and trust me, you need to see results. At first, I didn't see any betterment, and it was rather deflating. Jeffery showed me how to properly do what is known as the "Kegel" exercise to help with my incontinence. Listen, my friend, you will be doing these exercises all the time. I was doing them morning, noon, and night, and you will too, that is, if you want to see results! Kegel's involve tightening the muscles in your midsection which you use to stop the flow of urine, "the sphincter" muscles. It's quite simple. The easiest way I can describe how to do this exercise is to describe it like this. Perhaps a week before your surgery would be a good time to try these exercises. While in your restroom and standing in front of the toilet, you start your urine flow, just relax, let it flow naturally. Now, right after the midpoint of drainage, tightly squeeze your internal muscles (sphincters) and stop the urine stream from flowing out. Important: Do not try doing these at the beginning of your stream because the pressure will be too great at the beginning of the flow. Allow most of the fluids to come out and the pressure lowers to a point that you can be successful enough to stop the stream—that's it. Stopping the flow of urine is the Kegel exercise. It's that easy. Do this a couple of different times and you will get the basic knowledge. But don't do these Kegels while the catheter is in place. Importantly, after the catheter removal, don't do the midstream idea either. Wait 'til the drainage is completed and try a few right there at the toilet. It may be difficult on the first try, but keep trying each time you visit the restroom to urinate. Once you have done this a couple of times, you will get it right, and most importantly, you will feel the muscles getting stronger. A week later, try the midstream idea and see what happens. If you first can't stop the midstream, try at the end of the stream when pressure is the lowest, because it will be easier for you to stop the stream with lower pressure. Now, after you have discovered and mastered the correct way of performing the Kegel exercise, you can do them anytime, anywhere, during any part of the day. These Kegels aren't something you do just while urinating. Yes, at the start, only do them while at the toilet, because each time you perform a Kegel, a little urine will come out, and this way, the urine will drop securely into the toilet, not in your underwear. Doing them at the toilet is how you can know if you are doing them correctly. Correctly, it will shut off the flow of urine and push out a little urine at the end too. Once you have mastered the art of the Kegel exercise and your drips/squirts are ending, you can also do them while walking. You have to do this exercise day and night to be effective, but don't despair—they do work. Stopping your flow of urine after midstream is only to instruct you on how to do them correctly. That's not something you want to continuously do.

Now, for the second phase of Kegels. This is accomplished while you are standing at the toilet and after you have totally drained your antifreeze. Simply do ten or fifteen reps while still facing the toilet. It's easy. Squeeze for two seconds, relax for two seconds, and then just repeat the sequence for ten or fifteen reps each time you use the restroom. If you visit the restroom facilities five times a day, add it up. All right, I'll add it up for you. That's fifty Kegel exercises, and that's halfway to a hundred, which is the total reps you want to strive for every day. Do ten reps while you are sitting at the kitchen table. Do ten reps while watching TV during each commercial. When I'm watching a football game each time there is a long passing play, I'll do ten reps. If someone places you on hold while on the phone, do ten. While helping with the dishes, walking out to get the mail—use your imagination. I even exercise while walking through the grocery store with my wife and could easily do my 100 a day during one shopping trip. This is how I did it. While I was pushing the grocery cart down the different aisles, I would hold a Kegel while taking five steps and then release it and relax for ten steps. Again, I would hold it for five steps and release for ten steps. I kept repeating this technique throughout the store. Nobody would ever suspect a thing, and I get a good workout.

Here's a Budd note: You must ease into doing the Kegel exercises. The sphincter muscle is no different than any other body muscle. Start off slow and only do a few reps. No one starts off doing a hundred pushups. You start with five a day and then ten and work up over time. Same with these Kegels. After surgery, your body needs to heal. It has been through some trauma, so it's best to speak with your physician concerning the instructions on how to correctly do Kegels, how many to do, and ask how often to do them. If you are reading this and you have not already gone through the surgery yet, try doing some of these Kegels before it ever happens and get the hang of the process and how it works so that, afterward, you will already be up and running much like a hole shot at the drag strip.

And yet another Budd note: *Caution.* Do not do these Kegel exercises while the Foley catheter is in place. Practice them before surgery and after the catheter removal but not while the catheter is in place. Relax during the catheter time and only start after it has been removed. The 100 reps I mentioned earlier which I was doing while walking around the store, you must understand those 100 were not at the start of my doing Kegels. It was only after I worked up slowly to that amount. It was around six days after the removal that I made it to 100. After the months passed and the muscles got stronger, I actually did more than 100 per day. You certainly don't want to overuse these muscles at the start, so please be sure to get proper instructions from your doctor. Even now that it's been five years since my surgery, I still do these exercises every day.

I started slow, only fifty Kegels a day, and spread them out over the entire twenty-four-hour day. I started in the morning with my first visit to the restroom, and after doing my morning duty, I would complete five repetitions and continued doing five at different intervals throughout the day. After two days of working these muscles and seeing zero improvement and being a bit impatient, I bumped it up to sixty a day and stayed at sixty for two days and then moved to seventy-five a day. Before long, I was easily doing ten reps of ten a day. This was all new to me, and I desperately wanted to see improvement, but the reality is this process takes time. Every man is different. Keep going and doing all you can. Over time, you will see improvement. I did, and I was one of the worst-case scenarios you could read about. I found the best way for me to do the exercises was to hold each Kegel for three seconds and then release and relax for five seconds and then repeat for another round. Put your mind in the Kegel zone and do them periodically throughout the day. I was really striving to drive down the drips/leakage of urine because I had them pretty bad, worse than the normal guy. At this time, you should do a couple of things. First, doing the Kegel exercises consistently is the best thing. Second, cut back on the amount of fluid intake. I did the Kegel exercises like clockwork, not missing a beat, yet saw only minimal improvement which, again, was discouraging, and I even wanted to quit, but I knew better. I knew I couldn't quit. I wanted to be victorious of this thing.

The thing that made my slow improvement harder to understand was the stories of other guys who seemed to have way faster recoveries then me. Perhaps all the advertising material wanted to paint a prettier picture for all to read and didn't want to publish the latecomers or problem children like myself, and that's understandable. But still, I was a little disheartened. You may experience the same situation as I, but don't give in. It takes time, and believe me, it will work. I'm living proof because it took a long time for me and a lot of hard work. I was that poor guy at the bad end of the scale, the one nobody wants to talk about. I have come to the belief that it just takes time to build and train the nerves, the blood vessels, and these special muscles. I guess they don't respond as fast as, say, a bicep arm muscle. My advice is to be very patient with this part of the process. It was about a month before I could really say that there was a noticeable improvement and another two months before I noticed significant improvement. Not a stop to the problem, just improvement. Just don't give up or get discouraged, because that may start another unnecessary rollercoaster ride. By informing you of these types of situations throughout this book, my hope is that your rollercoaster rides are fewer. You will still surely have a few ups and downs because your journey will take you through unfamiliar territory. Completing my Kegels exercises at 100 a day as I did and also limiting my fluids showed me, over time, that my improvement was decent; however, it was not the end of my problem by any means, just a vast improvement, and for that, I was pleased, and that added an incentive to keep going forward, not looking back.

Like I said, I started out wearing man-type adult diaper underwear (I had no choice, I needed them, I honestly couldn't go without them). I have to pause for a moment here and put in a good report about these guys. They were discreet and provided me with protection. As much as I was leaking after the catheter was removed, I needed something, and these came in very handy and did their job. Of course, I changed a couple times each day for two reasons. One, I leaked a lot, and two, I was a neat freak (this cancer experience has lessened my neat freak attitude a little over the years in all phases of my life, and maybe for the better). As time progressed, I gained more control over my incontinence, and consequently, I graduated out of the adult underwear to wearing a product called Leak Guards. Thank God I found a friend to lean on called the "guards." I wore these guys inside my trunk-type underwear day and night, catching the drips which, I must tell you, wearing this stuff is a humbling experience and yet needful at the same time. My wife helped me a lot physically during my journey, and now she is helping me mentally. She is thankful that I am still around, and she will often tell me, "Honey, you're still here with me, and for that, I am grateful. We can deal with any leftover residue." She also said, "You made the right decision to eliminate it entirely." And I truly believe I did. Here's a Budd note: To maintain a positive outlook, you need to have positive people surround you.

Because of my ridiculous lack of control, I absolutely had to wear something to catch the unpredictable drips and those occasional and quite annoying tiny squirts. I was displeased with my lack of control, even though the drips and squirts were becoming less frequent, they were still happening. While growing up and working inside the construction arena, which I mentioned earlier, like all men, I developed a bit of a masculine outlook on life. This is where the story comes full circle. Big bad Budd was having trouble because he had to wear a diaper. Later, I had to wear a pad/leak guard in my underwear to catch uncontrollable drips. I was embarrassed, sort of like Samson getting his hair cut off. It was an embarrassing experience and an eye-opener. There will be aftermath problems no matter which procedure you choose. Believe me, they all have something that you will have to deal with. Every beautiful rose come with a thorn. They all have different problems with different scenarios and with different outcomes. Study all the information and talk with men who have gone through different procedures and ask them straight out about this problem, because you need to know the facts. The more types and different procedures you study, the better off you will be in choosing the one best for you. Do your homework and pick the treatment which best suits your life as it is now, in your present situation. Also, choose one that will be good for you in your future situations. Believe it or not, there are plenty of options out there, but you must search them out. They're not going to come around and be knocking on your front door.

I would like to interject something here about incontinence. There are several devices out there that claim to be great at helping with incontinence and/or the prevention of urinary leakage. Pay attention, brother, this is important; some of these devices are for stopping the urine from coming out, which should not be confused with products catching the urine as it comes out. Giant difference, my friend. My personal advice is don't use any of these external stopping devices, and always speak with you doctor before using anything at all. I'll tell you about some of the devices on the market. I'm not bad mouthing any of these devices, so no emails please. I am just saying, in my own opinion, I would not use them. Here is one device I believe is called the penile lock. It's a small device constructed in the shape of a U. It's a metal frame (some are plastic frame) and a foam rubber sponge-type material on the inside of the U. This device has a little clamp to hold the open end of the U closed after you have placed it onto your penis. Once you place this device onto your little hose, you begin to squeeze down on the clamp located at the opened end of the U shape which, in turn, squeezes down on the penis which, in turn, flattens the urethra which, in turn, prevents urine from leaking out. At first, it sounded pretty good and seemed fairly simple to use. It's the same action as taking a pair of vise clamp plyers and squeezing down on your backyard garden hose until the squeezing action completely stops the water from flowing out the far end of the hose. So at first sight, I said, "Hey, sounds OK. Why not use this theory on my own little personal garden hose?" But wait! Not so fast. I did some investigation on this device, and there are a few things I uncovered about the theory behind the way it works, which isn't so great, and of course, I am going to inform you about them right now.

1) If you squeeze down on your penis hard enough to stop the flow of urine, you might also be stopping the good flow of blood to vital areas. When you stop and begin to think rationally about how this device works, you honestly can't stop the urine flow without stopping some of the blood flow.

2) Now, if you leave this device on too long, you might be inadvertently be damaging yourself, and believe me, you do not want to damage your personal garden hose.

3) If you do use one of these devices and become dependent on it, then you are preventing yourself from ever having normal muscular control over the leaking. The easy way out is not always the best way out. So please, my brother, try to regain control over the leaking problem by your own physical muscles and mental abilities.

4) Question your doctor about any device (before using them), you might hear him say you should wait a certain length of time after surgery to use any sort of device, maybe up to eight months or longer, because he'll want you to get control over your problem the natural way and not with artificial devices. You are going to have to wait anyway for your body to heal, and you might as well use this healing time to practice Kegels and keep yourself safe.

5) Some men become dependent on these devices and end up skipping the Kegel exercises all together and remain incontinent. Not good, my friend.

6) Think about this. If you are artificially stopping the flow of urine, what's happening inside your body? I'll tell you what's happening. Your bladder is filling up and holding bile fluid inside of itself much longer than it knows it should (sometimes, our bodies are smarter than we are), and the holding-in for too long of this bile fluid can cause urinary infections. My doc always told me to get any human waste product out of the body quickly and completely. He told me, "Take the necessary time to totally drain the bladder before putting the pipeline back in your pants." Plus, with this artificial holding "U" clamp, whenever you remove the clamp, you better be ready, because if you held it too long, the dam is going to burst, and you may just spray all over the toilet or your pants. Cleanup time!

Here's a very simple and supportive tip I learned to help curb the drips/squirts and that I shall pass on to you: Urinate frequently. I have learned to not wait 'til I feel the urge to urinate. I know my own routine well enough now that if I have not gone for a while, I just mosey into the lavatory and drain any of my antifreeze that might be there. Like when I was a little boy, my mom would always tell me, "Go use the bathroom before we leave the house." Moms know things that we don't. I've learned to use the restroom before I set out on a shopping trip or before we head out for dinner or before going to the hardware store or, for that matter, wherever we are going. The last thing on my checklist is to hit the restroom on my way out the door. Halfway through a store or dinner, I'll use the restroom again. I named this practice, "Budd's frequent urinating routine." My means of using the word "frequent" doesn't equate to me having to go frequently. No, sir. Quite the opposite. It means I just use the restroom frequently and drain myself frequently. It's healthier too. Because I practice this method, when I do use the restroom, not a full amount of urine comes out at any one time, and, boss, that's "the key." If there isn't a lot of liquid in the bladder, then there isn't a lot of pressure inside the bladder, so consequently, there is less pressure to cause leakage. Frequent draining equals lower pressure which equals fewer drips. You should add this tip to all those notes your taking.

I was also advised by the same doc who said cut the fluids to avoid both caffeinated coffee and soda pop as another way to help cut down with my leaking issue. Presurgery, I went two weeks without tasting either one of those. It was easy, because even before surgery, I didn't drink very much of either one. Postsurgery, I went two months of abstaining from both items, and seeing that I was gaining more (not total, but more) control over the problem, I gradually introduced soda back into my intake of fluids. Only half a soda at a time, and only two days a week. I was very cautious. After a couple of weeks, I drank half a cup of coffee in the morning, drinking just a little at first to test the waters, like a small test campaign, if you will. I now have maybe two sodas a week and one full cup of my favorite caramel macchiato per week. I can't tell any difference from the time without them to the time with them, so I don't know if there was an influence from those two components for me one way or the other. This might be something you can try out for yourself. Maybe you will spot a difference. I think it may have to do with caffeine in those two items. Although, I have been told their effects on me may change as I age; however, as I age, I will continue to do the Kegels. Everyone is affected differently. Some doctors mainly suggest to avoid caffeine all together, so try different methods for yourself and find out which is better or worse. By simple deductive reasoning, you can eliminate what doesn't work and, of course, use that which does work.

Relax, sit back, and take a deep breath because there is light at the end of this tunnel and there's a lot of help out there to deal with incontinence. Be like me and just be glad to be alive. To be honest with you, at first, the drips and squirts were an enormous problem for me not just physically but mentally also. Everyone is different, and what might be difficult for me may be a breeze for someone else. Still, no matter what the problem is, time doesn't stop, the sun will always come up, and we all have to go on in life and deal with the problems that come against us. Remember, it's not the problems that come at you but how you deal with those problems. Find a solution, find a way around, over, or through the problem because you can bet your wallet there is a way out there. We only have this one life to experience, and the best thing to do is look at problems as opportunities to use all that gray matter inside your cranial vault. I'm not advocating that you go out and create problems. Just the opposite, because everyone knows problems seem to come enough by themselves; however, approach them with the positive attitude of being able to solve them and defeat them. After a while, you might find it fun to have victory over them. You might just become known as a "problem solver," which seems to be a man thing anyway.

For me, the problem of not being able to turn off the tap water was difficult to deal with, but I knew I had to keep working at it if I really wanted to see some progress, and man, I needed some real progress. I looked at a lot of different solutions, and I have to say, I tried most of them. From trying a variety of different pills that are on the market both from my doc and over the internet (which I must advise you not to do, at least 'til you speak with your doctor), to a whole new diet plan that helps, to a lot of salt, to a variety of different incontinence pads—from all-natural plans to the best artificial devices. The fact that there are so many options or so-called solutions and different philosophies out there to attack this problem told me something encouraging; it told me that I must not be the only man in the world facing this mountainous problem. Obviously, with so many so-called solutions out there, it must be a common problem which is not commonly talked about. Although, if it's such a common problem, why wasn't there more information for me in the books I read or perhaps more coming from the men I spoke with? Here are my thoughts on the problem. Perhaps it's because of slight embarrassment dealing with this issue and talking openly about it to others is taboo, or maybe some guys' experience with this problem wasn't so difficult. Perhaps they didn't have the same seriousness of the problem like I had. Mine was at the bad end of the scale. So if it was not as terrible for them, it meant they didn't even think about it. Possibly it may have to do with the fact that the absolute worst part of this continuous outflowing of fluids we men experience only last an average of about three to five weeks before we all begin to gain control over it and see significant improvement (mine, unfortunately, was much longer—one year long). Maybe because it is a short-term problem with some men, and perchance, some guys, for that very reason, don't feel it needs to be addressed in detail. Well, I'm addressing it for you right now in detail and in black and white.

For me, it was horrifying. At first, I had terrible thoughts of living with diaper rash for the rest of my life, and I didn't see an end to this problem. Cover-ups, yes; but an end, *no*. It was bad for me, and to be honest, some of the bad was due to me having a catheter in for twice as long and coupled with quite possibly that I was one of the unlucky ones who would have this problem for a long time and I was worse than the norm compared to most guys. I mean, there's always that one poor guy who has to be at the far end of the scale, and I seemed to be him. It's quite a humiliating situation to be in, because you can't escape it, not even for a couple hours; it's you, and you can't get away from yourself.

This next thought is funny. I thought up a neat little plan. I was going to make my own homemade outside catheter! This is what I was thinking. I could go to the hardware store, search for a very flexible two-foot long piece of tubing, which would, of course, actually fit over the end of my own personal hose and run it down my leg to a baggie at or around my calf muscle. In theory, this would work, but of course, it's just a Neanderthal-style catheter. Well, I didn't follow through with this idea, but I thought about it a lot because I was feeling so desperate, and I bet it would really work. It's probably good that I didn't follow through with this mad scientist idea, because I'm sure my beautiful wife would have had a few high-quality words for me if I had completed my folly thoughts.

I did investigate some other new things on the market. I say "new" because I didn't know about them before, so they were new to me, but some of the ideas are mainstream remedies for guys going through this. One item is adult undergarments. They are similar to the ones for toddlers, only larger, of course. Some even have elastic bands around the edges. I tried them because I was desperate, and the good news is they do work, and they work well, but there were two problems for me: (1) it would've taken me a long time to become accustomed to physically wearing them and also would have taken me a while to mentally get used to wearing them. I tried a couple of different types, and I will say they all worked quite well in dealing with the problem. (2) Even though they worked well, they didn't stop the problem, and stopping the problem is what I was looking for. I was trying to find something to stop the outflow or at least drastically slow it down. After some more investigating, I found a few other types of remedies of which some worked a little, some didn't work at all, and some, I honestly wouldn't even try.

Another therapy I read about was to consume more salt in my diet. The salt would act like a drying/water-absorption agent. What a giant myth this was. When I considered the amount of fluids which I personally was expelling compared to the amount of salt it was suggesting I ingest, I probably would have died from salt overdose before the water even dried up. Needless to say, I quickly moved on from this suggestion. I tried a few medications that proclaimed to solve the problem, and some of them actually helped. I will not mention their names here, but one is a familiar decongestant—your doctor will tell you about it. A few other treatment options for incontinence are internal collection devices, an artificial urinary sphincter, an external device called a condom catheter which, funny enough, is a little like my homemade Neanderthal catheter idea. Some doctors offer collagen injections. That's an idea I would not even try but is highly advertised. I even investigated one treatment called "electrical stimulation." A surgical treatment called a "male sling." If you ask your urologist, they might rattle off a couple more options for you to try. Just investigate any treatment option copiously, get several opinions from completely different sources, not two doctors who work together but competitors who will offer different and opposing viewpoints, do your homework, and find the right solution for your situation. Your doc will help you too.

To be quite honest with you, all the different medications, including the decongestant, did a satisfactory job of "helping" me dry out while the other items helped in keeping me dry, but none ended my situation; they only helped, and all along, I still continuously practiced my Kegels. I really wasn't wanting any artificial devices, and I am definitely not up for surgical treatments, and again, this advice is only mine and my way of thinking. There are different scenarios for different men in different situations. My incontinence (while I may have thought was horrible) is not at the point to take any of the above drastic steps like surgery. If it was, I might be singing a different tune to you right now. All the things I tried certainly didn't fix my problem, but I have to say, some of them did help, and I was grateful for any help. The single major item to help with my incontinence, which was with me all along, just like Dorothy's ruby slippers—she carried them with her all along—was simple, I had to do a lot of good old-fashioned physical Kegel exercises and penile rehab. One side note to interject here: I couldn't handle some of the side effects from some of the different medications. Some side effects are as bad as the problem they are trying to fix. Now, because of my career in construction and the amount of heavy lifting required in that field of work, I experienced lower back problems on and off the job site and became very familiar with back pain. One of the side effects from a couple of different pills was a slow nagging backache right around the lower kidney area, which I didn't like. Although the meds helped with the drips, I put them aside, and this is why: In reality, I was trading one problem for another problem. Plus, I don't like ingesting a lot of different medication. I'm just big on the natural way of things.

It's unfortunate to say, but sometimes, some of the prescription medications are as difficult to deal with as some of the conditions they are trying to treat. Here's a funny spot. One doctor said he could prescribe another med to counter the side effects of the first pill, so now I would be taking two pills—it's not me. I was busy searching for that elusive magical potion over the months with few true results. Another side note for you; throughout the months of time that I was searching for that magical potion, I kept on diligently performing those Kegel exercises which I was instructed to do by the good doc Jeffery in the very beginning, and because of my diligence with these Kegel exercises and the reduction of fluids, I did notice improvement within my state of affairs from my own actions. I wish I could tell you within these pages that I found that magic tonic and actually pass that information onto you, but alas, there is no such magical tonic. A lot of diligent physical work in practicing the Kegels, drinking the lower appropriate amount of liquid, exercising rehab, and a little bit of luck seem to be the real mystical tonic.

As I was saying, the dripping problem was starting to subside as time continued. I didn't say it stopped. The problem was still there and still an issue for me to deal with, it just wasn't as wicked as it was in the beginning. Throughout my journey, I must tell you that I found one product that helped me the best. They were almost, not quite, but close to being worry-free, quite easy to use, had odor control, very discreet, and were not visible. My problem—little drips which, by the way, were slowing down in frequency. Since I couldn't stop them yet, I turned to absorbency as the key factor for help and consideration at this time until I could get physical control over the drips. For me, these little guards helped fit the bill immensely. Most guys will understand when I say they fit like an athletic cup. At this time, the leak guards really came to my rescue. I finally found an able partner in the fight against the drips, and I shall readily advise you to get a pack of these little helpers.

I'll let you in on a little secret about those drips. About 50 percent of the time, you can't even feel them coming out. They're seem to be quite clever about waiting 'til the coast is clear and then sneaking out undetected and then turning around and laughing at you. They remind me of myself when I was a teenager and living at home. Occasionally, you can feel them as they are escaping because you can physically feel them course through the end your penis. You may just need to lift something or move a heavy object and you'll feel them. However, for the rest of the time, you won't feel these little guys escaping at all.

While doing a lot of walking, such as walking around inside a large store or at the mall, looking at different items, contemplating what to purchase, my mind would be busy on other matters such as the products on my shopping list and not paying attention to the little drips that would be sneaking out and into my underwear, but after a while, I could feel the dampness that they caused, but not anymore. Thank heavens for my new partner—the leak guard. It was an essential assistant, and I'll now endorse them for your use. The leak guard apprehends the drips and squirts as they seem to merrily come out and into the open. But not now, my little drips. Ha-ha! My leak guard gobbles them up instantly, much like the old video game I played called *Pac-man*. The guard absorbs them and holds them tight and safely until you can get to a restroom. The guard is on duty for your safety the entire time you use them and happily gobbles any drips while you can cheerfully continue with what you're doing. My life became easier. As I said earlier, the problem seemed to be the amount of drips that were escaping even though they seemed to be decreasing weekly. Since I couldn't stop the problem, I turned to being able to control them, and these guards were a huge help. I changed the leak guard every three hours and could even go for longer periods as my journey continued onward and my control grew better. Now, because I have such good control, one guard would last me all day if I needed it to. Thanks to the good lord for that. A small hint: Do not flush these guards down the toilet. Place them in the trash can.

Believe me, I understand why these leak guards for men are sold in large packages, and I purchase the ones containing fifty-two leak guards. Man, in the very beginning, when I first found these little helpers, I was so thankful for them. I was going through about five guards a day. That equals one package every eleven days—too much, too fast, too often. I concluded that I was changing them too frequently. I've been accused of being a neat freak, and of course, I was checking them throughout the day and was not familiar with their absorbency or their efficiency, which meant when I would check and see that it had gathered some of my drips (and was grateful for their gathering), I would take it off and place a new one in its place. Well, in truth, I was just changing the leak guard more than was needed. Those guards were engineered to absorb far more than I was allowing them to. However, after I completely blazed through the first fifty-two pack of guards, my lightning-fast mind began understanding their efficiency, and my frequent changing habit slowed way down, I mean like down to two pads a day, which extended my guards to a month for the fifty-two-pack which is much improved. It was an immense difference after I realized what they were capable of doing. Now, I can honestly tell you right here that, because of my control, one pack of these will last two months easily (yahoo) and the reason is I only need one if I will be doing a lot of walking around, such as if I was going Christmas shopping or if I was going over to my buddy's place to help him work on his house.

Another small hint for you, "cargo pants," because you will need to carry a spare guard on your body while going on a visit of four hours or more.

I truly hope that by reading my stories and getting a better understanding of the pitfalls I went through, the information in this book may help you through your journey. The fewer rollercoaster rides, the better. No one understands the hazards of any journey unless they have walked the path themselves, so if you are just starting out, then I'm hoping to help you have an easier path to walk.

As I said, the leak guards were a great helper, and I continued with my Kegel exercising. I did those Kegels religiously every day and all day. Although, to be honest with you, as time went on, I became a bit more panicked that perhaps this leaking situation was going to be my normal new way of life (another rollercoaster). That very thought was disturbing to me. My doctors were very helpful and supportive from the actual start of my journey, but they are busy men and have many patients to deal with; they can't always babysit everyone.

As you read the next sentence, I'm asking that you not judge me too harshly. I understand it's going to sound like I'm rather vain, but here goes. I found myself being quite embarrassed as I was standing in the checkout lane at the grocery store and watching the clerk grab hold of the bag of Depends for Men (manufactured by Kimberly-Clark) and run it over the machine to scan the code on the package and then watching it pass by me on the moving belt and into the hands of the bagger, who pushes it off to the side because it's too big to fit into the plastic bags the store provides. The one positive mental note throughout this checkout lane experience, coupled with the associated wearing of the guards all day, is that it gave me a far healthier appreciation, and a new admiration, for the women in my life. I mean, God bless the women of this world, they have dealt with these products almost on a daily basis for the best part of their lives. Myself, I just started these products, and it was all new to me. I mean, before this, I was totally oblivious to what women go through. I never really gave it much thought, and I know why. I'm a guy, and it didn't directly affect me, so it never registered inside my big lug head, and for that, I must apologize. You see, for years, while I would be standing alongside my wife in the checkout lane, watching her purchase the many various packages of feminine products with different colors, different styles, and sizes for different needs. I never once gave a thought about the time or inconvenience and the huge hassle it must be to her and for that matter all females. It suddenly opened up a new respect and understanding for her, because seeing it now represented all the time, effort, and everything else a woman must go through. Now I know, now I understand, and you ladies have my sympathy and my request for forgiveness.

Newsflash! The day my outlook changed concerning the man pads. In all honesty, as I said before, I was embarrassed standing in line at the grocery store and purchasing a bag of them. My wonderful soulmate told me something that fired up a lightbulb inside my Neanderthal mind and changed my whole outlook on these pads with only a few simple words of wisdom from her. She basically told me that these items I was now purchasing and wearing are not *pads*. She said they're not even called pads, they don't look like pads, and they're not labeled anywhere on the package as pads, so listen up, ya big lug nut, you need to stop calling them pads. She said to look at the package and read the label. They're called *guards for men*. Wow— that was mind-blowing. Once again, the woman was right. I never really contemplated how they were label before. It seemed to ease my mind when I realized that these aren't pads at all and nowhere on the package did it even mention that word. I was looking at this with the wrong perspective and the wrong attitude. It's called a guard, and it's for men, it performs a function, it does a job for me, it guards me from dealing with damp underwear, it guards me from embarrassment, it helps me, it protects me. Wow, plus the word "guard" sounded way better than pad. From that point forward, my perspective changed.

Now, on a lighter note, here's a Budd nugget of information on underwear for us guys. Boxer shorts became nonexistent for me. I mean, you have to securely keep these guards in their strategic location so they can do their job accurately. I discovered for myself that boxer shorts fit too loose and could not hold the guard securely in place. So I moved on from boxers and tried a couple pairs of tight-fitting briefs. Although the briefs fit well and worked fine in conjunction with the leak guards, you all know me well enough by now that I still wanted to experiment with other styles, and one style I wore years ago turned out to be the best for holding the guard in place and were the most comfortable—they're called "trunks." If you're one of those guys who don't care for the brief-style underwear, try the trunk style. I found they were the best fitting with the best overall performance of comfort and holding skill. They're actually just like tighter fitting boxer shorts anyway, and you can always return to your style of underwear once things are under control and you have no need for wearing the leak guards. The trunk style fits snug and holds the guard in the proper place while holding all your personal goodies in their respective places.

I'm going to reiterate that making more frequent visits to the restroom is also a must; the muscles which hold in the body's urine are not what they used to be. They will be stronger in the future, but right now, not so much, so even if your physical half isn't informing you that you have to urinate, your mental half should be telling you to go drain your antifreeze. Draining your bladder many times throughout the day and predominantly just before retiring for the night is preventive maintenance. This is because your sphincter muscles are unable to hold the volume of urine in the bladder at this particular time, not like they could prior to the surgery. The good news is the muscles will be able to hold more volume as time goes on. You, and only you, must strengthen those muscles. Like I said earlier, there is no Dumbledore wizard waving his wand to create a magic potion. The bladder is constantly accumulating urine from your kidneys twenty-four hours a day, drip by drip, and over the hours, it does add up. Multiple trips to the restroom will drain this buildup which, in turn, produces less dripping. Every guy performs preventive maintenance on their car. Only now, bro, it's preventive maintenance on your body. Just like your car, you are doing this to help prevent problems later.

You'll be happy to find one very big milestone as you continue further into your recovery journey, and it comes when you do not have to wear a guard throughout the night. I was absolutely elated when I reached this point. In fact, it was a hallelujah moment for me. It's a small step forward in the grand scheme of things, yet it was another giant leap forward for Buddkind. Two different forces come together while you are sleeping:

Force #1. if you have been doing your Kegel exercises regularly, your internal urinary control muscles, which have control over the outflow of urine and bladder control, will become stronger, which helps in stopping the drips. These internal muscles are two different groups located at two different places, and both are called sphincter muscles (one called internal, one called external). These groups of muscles are the target of those Kegel exercises you will be doing. Every time you do a Kegel, you are strengthening these muscles a little further, and they become a little stronger which, in turn, means they perform a better job of closing the urethra and thus stopping the flow of urine.

Listen up, my dear friend, because I am telling you something. Here's the key to unlock the door of the recovery process. If you do the Kegel exercises correctly and diligently and you energize these sphincter muscles so they become strong enough to completely close off the urethra all by themselves, then you don't need the medicines, the pills, the devices, or the guards. Another way to help the entire area all around the sphincter muscles is an exercise for men. Lay down on your back, on the carpet, with your knees up and feet toward your butt. Now, raise your midsection off the floor.

The way I understand it, one group of sphincter muscles is located just above our prostate gland at the base of the bladder. The second group is located below the prostate gland. These two sphincter muscle groups encircle the membranous urethra exactly like the donut-shaped prostate gland does. The urethra, as described previously, is essentially a long spherical-shaped tube that urine flows through in order to exit the body. The length of this tube leisurely winds its way from the base of the bladder down through the first set of sphincter muscles, continues straight through the middle of the prostate, enters the second set of sphincter muscles, and continues its way straight through the center of the penis and out the tip. Our urine travels all that distance just so it can splash merrily into the toilet.

Force #2. The second force that happens while sleeping through the night is the body's position. You are laying down. It's simple physics again. Gravity tells water to always seek out the lowest point and run to it. It's why you always see streams and rivers running downhill and, eventually, to the ocean. You will never see water running uphill by itself; it is against the laws of physics (which is basically Mother Nature, and we all know not to cross our moms). Well, inside all of us guys, there is a small stream, and it wants to run downhill 'til it exits our bodies and splashes into the toilet, which is sort of like the ocean for our urine. When a man is standing upright, his lowest point would be—you guessed it. When you are lying down on the bed, usually on your back, all the pipelines run horizontal; gravity cannot work its magic. So while in this position, you are helping yourself to stop the flow, which stops the drips. In some small way, you could say you have overcome the force of gravity. For me, when I reached the point of no guards during the night, I was very happy. In fact, I did a little happy dance right there in the bedroom where my enthusiasm was quickly extinguished by a few little drips. I still had to wear the leak guards during the day (gravity again), but reaching this point of not wearing them at night was quite a milestone for my journey.

As time went on, it was extremely cool not needing the guard at night, which was a point of progress. I'm sure it will be for you too. After a couple more months, I realized that all those Kegel exercises were beginning to pay some dividends back to me. I was progressing to the point where I didn't need a guard when I first got out of bed in the morning. Now this morning thing was another significant eye-opener for me and just one more hallelujah moment. Soon as I awoke in the morning, I would scurry over to the restroom to drain my overnight accumulation of antifreeze. Plus, after totally draining my stuff and while still standing at the toilet, I would do about twenty Kegels. Yes, you heard me correctly—Kegels at the toilet.

Get out your pencil and paper, this next one is good. This idea came to me one morning, and it worked so well I continued with the practice. Kegels are a must-do, and it's actually very convenient to do them while standing at the toilet. Here's a Budd fact: When a guy is practicing his Kegel exercise, the simple act of doing them may produce several mini squirts of urine or at least a few drops, so standing at the toilet, the squirts and drips can conveniently drop right into the water. Anytime during the day you find yourself standing (or sitting) at the toilet, you will discover this is a textbook opportunity to be "tinkling and kegeling." Sounds like a country western song title! But on the serious side, doing at least ten or twenty Kegels at this time can give you a tremendous advantage in the mornings. Also, think about this—you should be using the restroom to drain your bladder more frequently during your journey to aid in combating the dreaded drips, and while doing these frequent trips to the restroom during the day, you should be doing ten Kegels right there at the toilet. Excellent timing, you're now multi-tasking. Remember, five trips to the restroom during the day, and you're halfway to the 100 per day mark. Always check with your doctor on their recommendations on the amount and frequency of performing Kegels, because it will change as time goes by. At first, take it easy building those muscles slowly and properly, and then, as your sphincters get stronger, you can place the pedal to the metal and begin to rev up the RPMs to hit the 100-plus mark. The 100-a-day mark was my absolute minimum amount to complete over the course of every twenty-four-hour day, and I still strive for that mark today.

As I mentioned in the last paragraph, when I recognized the little bit of morning progress I was making, it really put a smile on my face and made me want to do even more Kegels. At first, not wearing a guard at night and also for a short period of time in the mornings was something I counted as a good thing, and that progress provided much needed encouragement for me to continue to achieve my goals. I truly hope that your recovery is short. As time continued, the length of time of not wearing the guard lengthened. After one more month, I noticed I could go about two hours in the morning without wearing one. It was almost an entire year before I reached the point of not having to wear one during the morning hours. I'm not going to sugarcoat this; my recovery took a long time. It was slow and it's a reality you may have to live with also, but let's look at the bright side here. Let's really hope you are one of the luckier ones and it takes less time for you, but don't get discouraged if you don't see results immediately. The truth is, it may not happen, but here's a wonderful thought: With the continuing progress of medical science, the medical surgeons should be able to do a better job in today's world now more than ever before. Medical advancements happening today are tipping the scales in your favor, so your recovery will not only be assured but also shorter.

So now, back to the poor guy at the end of the scale—that's me. While not needing a guard at night and almost until noon the next day was great, I still wore one during the largest part of my waking hours and especially if I would be doing a lot of walking, but I was diligently watching and recognizing my progress and so should you. Not wearing one until noon was an advancement in my journey.

My Ideas on Wearing and Changing of the Guard Part 1—"Wearing"

Here's a tip you can write in your notebook. Again, nobody informed me of this. I figured it out on my own, and I'm hoping it will help you too. How to wear the guard and how to change it. You want to keep the guard in place with a snug fit. Think of this guard as another piece of your own clothing or more precisely a piece of your personal insurance clothing. Guards need to be held in place securely, and the best way to accomplish this small achievement is to wear a snug fitting pair of undershorts; otherwise, it will shift out of place. I'm telling you straight up, boss, if the guard slips out of place, your underwear gets wet, and you'll be embarrassed. Something else, my friend, if it isn't held in place securely, you may find yourself constantly adjusting its position within your shorts and your constant adjusting will look inappropriate, especially if you find yourself adjusting this guard while walking down the food aisle at the grocery store, which can be embarrassing, especially if the security guard comes up to you and wants to know why you are walking through the store with your hands down your pants.

Speaking about being embarrassed, I'll enlighten you with a short story of an unfortunate, uncomfortable, and embarrassing incident from the life of Budd. It starts in our home. It's a beautiful mid-July day. Sunny outside as well as inside my heart, because I love nice warm weather. After eating breakfast, I made my usual half-gallon of sweet tea. By noon, I had maybe four glasses of my special tea in my favorite fourteen-ounce frosted mug which, in hindsight, was my first mistake of the day, because it's an overdose of liquids in such a short period of time. I was in our kitchen placing more ice in my glass when my wife walked in. She wanted to go to Target. She had a few coupons for paper towels and wanted to use the coupons before their expiration date, and while at the store, she wanted to stock up on other household essentials. My wife is good at making our house a home. Anyhow, I said, "Lets' roll. I'll drive." I took one more long drink of tea, hit the restroom, scooped up the car keys, and made our way to the store. We're in the store, and at this point of the story, we've been gone about an hour, had most of our stocking goods, and were almost done with our shopping. I was wearing a pair of light khaki shorts. My wife was pushing the cart and was just a few steps in front of me. She stopped, turned around to ask me a question, and *wham-o!* One hand goes over her mouth and her other hand points right to the middle section of my shorts. There it was, front and center—a wet spot the size of a golf ball. That's what you call instant embarrassment!

Here's the thing, while walking around, you may not feel the drips as they come out. If you're walking fast or jogging, you won't feel them at all. The positive things about the leak guards is that they perform their job really well as long as they are held in place properly and securely. Their good performance means you may not always be aware of how damp or wet the guard may actually be during the day. You should visibly check your guard and also still visit the restroom often (my second mistake was not using the restrooms at the store midway through). You don't want yourself to be caught off guard (no pun intended). This is the kind of information no one tells anyone about, but we all need to know. You may not always hear some of this info from the doctors or other gents you speak with. Doctors are not going to spend hours going over details. Some things are going to be up to you. To us guys going through this time, it's a big deal, not a small detail. Plus, if the docs themselves have not gone through this journey, they may not even know these details. I found all these details out myself simply through trial and error, and I hope these stories enlighten you for your help. Maybe you won't have to go through some of these if you learn from my mistakes.

My first mistake in this story was drinking too much liquid too fast. My second mistake was not hitting the restroom for one of my frequent draining's. My third mistake was not double-checking the fitting of the guard, which I should have, because this day, I was not wearing my snug-fitting trunk-type underwear. I was wearing an older pair of underwear, and the guard shifted just enough to create a breach in the system. As soon as I returned home, I took off the old pair of underwear and tossed them in the trash. I promised myself that little embarrassing mishap would never happen again.

Wearing and Changing of the Guard Part 2

"Changing" of the guard will be something of a personal preference. I feel it is my obligation to suggest that you change the guard often, particularly in the beginning of your journey and then slow down. The first reason to change often is simply for you to get to know the performance of the guards: how they work, how much they can absorb, and how fast they absorb it, or in other words, how long can you go 'til you say enough is enough and then have to change it. Just don't go to long on your first couple of tries, because it can be a little awkward. Learn what works for you and what works for the guard.

The second reason to change is for your personal hygiene. They drier you are and the drier the guard is, the fewer bacteria there are. We are all aware of the pain an infant goes through when they develop diaper rash; we don't want that here. Another tiny reason for frequent changing is that human urine has a very unique one-of-a-kind scent. It can turn embarrassing if you are standing around talking with a group of people and you notice one of them sniffing the air. They may have a strange look on their face reflecting that they know what the odor is but can't seem to find where it's coming from, that is, until you leave the group.

In the very beginning, I honestly decided to change my guard numerous times a day, but that's only because I was a neat freak. Multiple changing made me feel far more comfortable. I discovered that changing times can vary; it depends of a couple of things. It may depend on the amount of fluid one consumes during the day. More fluids obviously mean more drips, and the more drips/squirts mean frequent changing of the guard. Another thing is more frequent trips to the restroom will tremendously help with fewer changing of the guards. If you don't keep up with the timely excursions to the restroom and you pick up something heavy, you will feel a squirt. After a few squirts, you better check your personal area because you may need to change the guard. The more Kegels you perform, the more control you will have over the drips, and that, again, will change the situation. If you are one of the lucky gentlemen and your problem is hardly noticeable, one guard might last you all day. I'm sure after a week or so of your own trial and error, it shall be obvious to you when you need to change and you will settle into a routine and be OK with it. Remember, the stronger the sphincter muscles, the fewer the drips.

CHAPTER 8

Erectile Dysfunction (ED)

You might also be dealing with just a touch of erectile dysfunction, also known as impotence. This ED issue can be caused by several things such as low blood flow into the penis and/or damage to the nerves that control erections. There are more reasons too, but they get into medical disorders, atherosclerosis, and also ingesting different types of medications; however, we don't need to go there because we are only speaking about the first two I mentioned above—low blood flow within the blood vessels that supply the penis and perhaps damage to the surrounding nerves.

I found, during my time of decision making, there were very few exceptions within the many available different treatment options with this type of cancer that does not have some effect on the ability to have an erection or some other side effect connected with ED. Damage may be done to the surrounding nerves and/or blood vessels which aid in the ability to get an erection and also maintain an erection. The brain and hormones still work with all their intensity, but damage to the blood vessels and/or tiny nerves can occur with removal of the prostate and other types of treatments. Nerves and blood vessels are very slow to heal, but in most cases, they can heal. In my case, I couldn't manufacture an erection for about six months, and in the seventh month, things slowly improved; however, it was far from the erections I was accustomed to, and unhappily, the erections I finally was able to achieve weren't nearly as hard as they were before, which meant I was unable to penetrate. This is a serious let-down for any man, and I know it was a bit of a letdown for my wife, although she never said a negative word about it. Whatever hardness there was tended not to last very long. I have to say, I was very sad, disheartened, and disappointed. My wife would tell me, "It doesn't matter. At least I still have you with me." She supported the decision to rid myself of that monster, and if this is one thing we needed to work on, then let's do the work and so be it.

My doc instructed me to prepare for what is known as "penile rehab." Now, as I'm writing these words down on paper, "penile rehab" sounds odd and also kind of humorous. I mean really, rehab for the little guy. When I was younger, he never took a day off. We tried the rehab, and of course, during the time I was doing the rehab, I must say it wasn't humorous at all. True, yes; humorous, no.

Prior to surgery, I was a typical guy: I would get an erection hard enough to hang a bath towel on and then jump around the room beating my chest like a gorilla in the zoo. After the surgery, I swear it was exactly like a wet noodle. I mean, literally, it was as different as night and day. I probably could have tied it in a knot like a shoestring. For months, we worked on the penile rehab and used the pills my doctor instructed us to and tried some others that were available on the market for some help, but sad to say, nothing really worked. Plus, low back aches came with those meds and the occasional headache. I once more had my rollercoaster thoughts, which would be normal for any guy, mostly because I was worried it may never work again; it didn't look like it was ever going to work again, and just being honest here, my little friend right now wasn't working at all. Also adding to the rollercoaster ride was the fact that some of the literature I read was frightening since it had a small percentage of men stating within the literature that they never regained their ability to have an erection. My doc was quite positive and reaffirmed me many times.

He said, "Budd, we get better at this stuff every day. Don't despair. This takes time." He also stated that "it's not uncommon for some men to take a year or possibly even a little longer to come back, but it will happen for you." Nevertheless, he assured me it would heal properly. It does take time, and I might add, it does take "work" on your part.

Now, I'm sure you probably just stopped reading and started asking yourself, "What does Budd mean when he said it takes work on your part?" My good doctor Jeffery instructed my wife and myself on the work it takes, and I'll pass his advice onto you. First, he said we must be patient and let things heal, put in the time and the work it will take, try diffident meds, and you must try exercising the little guy with penile rehabilitation, which basically means eye and hand stimulation every couple of days, which also means we have to physically stimulate the penis so blood will begin to flow through the blood vessels within the area which makes it hard and to help the nerves grow back and slowly heal all the parts that are hurting. Talk about taking matters into your own hands.

Talk with your doctor about penile rehabilitation and any medications that may help. It took me a long, long, long time; however, it does work. It takes patience, perseverance, and hard work (that's not a pun). There are many testimonials where men tell their stories, and it only took them three months to recover and no use of drugs, which would have been wonderful if that would have happened to me, but sadly no. Another gentleman's testimonial said six months before he was back to normal—not my luck. With me, it was a year, and I can assure you it was a long year. I hope that you will be one of the many gentlemen with good results and faster results than myself. Plus, with medical advances, your chances grow better every minute. The doc will tell you when to do and how to do the rehab, and there are many other avenues to go down to find help during the rehab e.g., medications that can be prescribed for you such as Viagra, Levitra, or Cialis. These meds can all aid in the recovery process. Each man is different. Try each med and record the differences between them so you will be aware and be able to use the best one for yourself.

Levitra and Viagra are closely related in the way they work. You take them about forty minutes before need them and they will continue to work for around five hours. Cialis is a little different. You take it about three hours before you need it, and its effects can last up to thirty-six hours. However, as you read what I'm writing, please don't take it as the absolute gospel, times change, advancements happen, medicine changes, so you should always consult your own person physician.

I was given a couple of different medications to try and help with the ED, but Cialis was the one that helped me the most with the least amount of side effects. It was in my seventh month before I ever felt it getting stiff—not hard by any stretch of the imagination. In my eighth month, I actually felt it was getting close to being hard which, I might add, put a smile on both of our faces because it was progress but, unfortunately, still not hard enough to penetrate, and believe me, we tried. Each time my wife would get it somewhat hard and we would give it a try, the little guy just bent to the side and wouldn't penetrate. Believe me, it was so disappointing that any stiffness that was present just seemed to melt away, partly because, mentally, it was a giant letdown to me and, of course, inside my head, I would begin to think that I was also letting down my wife. I think I was at the brink of giving up, and at those low moments inside your journey, please don't give in to those thoughts—I almost did. I found that perseverance is the key, and my wife was right by my side to encourage me on.

It was approximately one lengthy year before I was able to become hard enough to penetrate. My wife and I were able to make love and enjoy that wonderful satisfaction. When that moment did finally happen, I really did beat my chest and jump around the room like a gorilla but still couldn't hang a towel on it, but no matter, being able to penetrate was another big milestone in my journey. Looking back twelve months earlier when I didn't think my little buddy was going to come back to life because, believe me, it wasn't getting hard at all, I was beginning to be totally saddened with thoughts of the aspect of living with this problem the rest of my life and never getting back to normal. So I can tell you, when you get down or discouraged, remember, I was there also; in fact, many others before us have been there too. Please listen to the doctors telling you that it will be OK. It will happen. Read my words, it will come back, it takes time and a lot of rehab work, but maybe, just maybe, you could be one of the lucky ones where it only takes a few months not a full year like myself, and if so, count your blessings, brother. Therefore, at those times when, to you, it may look and feel hopeless on your end, just try to remember what others are telling you. Take hope in their words and don't fall into the negative despair pit. It took me a year to come back, and yes, I won't lie, there was despair and even some anger at different times of the journey on my behalf, but let me clarify what I'm saying and perchance these words will give you hope. It's OK if, at times, you do have despair—we all do at some time or another—but don't let the gloom rule. Don't let it win.

Think of it this way, the method you use to not let the despair win is to not dwell on it. As with anything in life, don't live in the negative. Understand it's there but think of how you can beat it. Think of yourself as being victorious. See yourself with a couple of scars that are, in reality, lifelong medals of honor given to you by life itself because you won the battle—you beat a menacing monster cancer. I'm saying pick yourself up and look despair in the eye. Understand it happens but then turn around and put equal effort into looking at the good side. Spend more time looking at the positive side. Look to the hope that all will turn out fine and dandy in the end. Look at the fact that you are still here. Some guys didn't make it. Paul didn't. You are blessed to be living. That's big. It may take time, but see the good light at the end of the tunnel, and once again, that is where you have to look. Don't look at where you are now inside the tunnel but focus on the light at the end of the tunnel because that, my friend, is the goal of this journey. Keep your eyes and your faith looking forward, not down at your feet. Look at everything as motivation for yourself to become victorious.

OK, I stated it was a year before I was back to normal. Although, to be honest with you, I wasn't all the way back to normal, it was a year after my surgery, but I wasn't back to 100 percent normal. When a person gets one of those devastating phone calls then journeys through cancer treatments like this one or, for that matter, any cancer treatment, believe me, you are never going to be back to the before normal self. You have to find a new normal, and it's a little different than the old normal. Sure, other people may be looking at you because they see the outside and they may think you are back to normal, but on the inside, not so much. Psychologically and physiologically, you have been altered.

It was a great improvement and a huge milestone for me just to be hard enough to penetrate and have an intimate and personal time with the woman I love. Being at 90 percent of my normal is still a huge percentage, and my wife was thankful too. Now after several more years have passed, I would rate my normal as 95 percent.

However, I stated earlier that I wasn't going to sugarcoat anything. I also stated I would explain everything that happened to me during my journey. Here goes another piece of my puzzle within my personal situation concerning my journey and a special thing I feel compelled to educate you on. Now, this one thing I'm about to explain was for me and still is of no consequence to me, because in my life, I wasn't desiring any more children and I also truly wanted that cancerous enemy completely eliminated and out of my body, but it might be something to be considered by you. Here is an explanation of our prostate glands' main purpose.

Our prostate glands main goal for being inside the male body is to aid in the reproductive process. Once our gland is removed, there will be no more reproductive process. In other words, there will be no reproducing fluids coming out of your body. No fluids, no children. You should consult with the doctor about this. I'm sure he'll give you a better rendition than I just did, but I'll try to explain it to you the best I can. Our gland is a mixing station. It brings together and introduces the necessary fluids to our sperm and then pumps both into our pipeline (the urethra) as they blend together and begin their own journey out of our body. Without the prostate gland being in place to propagate this mixing process and also injecting these fluids into our pipeline, these fluids will not make it into the urethra pipeline, so naturally, they will not be coming out either. I didn't fully understand this concept when it was explained to me in the very beginning of my journey, and if you don't comprehend it right now either, well, it's OK, but I will, however, try and explain it a little further for you in a slightly different way.

Here's goes. We, as men, have been through this cycle many, many, many times during our lives. We first get mentally excited which, in turn, makes blood begin to be pumped into the penis and we begin to get hard, and then it proceeds to become an erection which then continues on to the point of orgasm. At orgasm (our climax), the fluids and sperm are being mixed together. This mixture is then injected into our urethra pipeline, where it's quite happily ejected out and into the universe. Well, after the prostate is removed, the process changes a bit from the normal. At first, it's still pretty much the same; we get mentally excited and we begin to get hard and then it proceeds to become an erection which, then again, continues on to the point of orgasm. It all feels the same and looks the same. However, at climax, this is the point of change. Nothing comes out, no sperm is ejected. All the emotions are there, all the highs are there, all the correct action is there, but no sperm is there. It's as if the fluids are all in the same car, they're on the right highway and headed to the city, but they take the last exit ramp before entering the city. At first, it was all quite strange to me, almost like I was missing out on something, and of course, I was. Like I stated earlier, I will usually try to look at the good in any situation, and I have to say, I learned, in some cases, this may be a very positive attribute. Well, I got off-track again like I always do; however, the above is some important information that I believed you should be aware of. It might help you in the decision process. It did for me because I no longer wanted to father offspring.

Now back to the topic of our previous conversation which is "ED." Believe me, during my first twelve months, I tried a variety of different solutions with tenuous results. Some worked mildly, and some didn't work at all. I must say to you, in retrospect, that I was perhaps trying too hard or possibly trying to do too much or even trying to make it work too fast, and of course, that lead to more mental disappointment and a couple of those rides I don't like. All bodily healing does take time (especially nerve damage and may take twelve months to heal and will need intense physical therapy), and possibly, I should have relaxed a little and just let all things work out naturally, because for me, everything seems to take a long time anyway, no matter what I did. Think about my journey. It took a long time for me to even set up a physical with my general practitioner a.k.a. "primary care doctor" who actually started me down this journey. After those few visits, it took a long time for all the pieces of my journey to come together. It took a couple of years for the urologist to see all the intricate pieces and different things beginning to line up, it took a long time for me to gather up the information for me to make my decision, it took twice the normal time to remove the catheter, it took a long time to stop the drips, and at last, it took a long time me to come back from impotency, so perchance, it was just my fate that each part of my life and my journey played out as it did, and of course, continuing on, it took me a long time to write this book.

During my long months of penile rehab (which sounds amusing now), the one thing I did not like was taking the different medications. I've never been a fan of taking a lot of different prescription drugs; besides, I really lean toward the natural way of doing things. However, this is the twenty-first century, which means science and medicine are at its pinnacle of technology. I'm smart enough to know that, sometimes, with somethings within our lives here on earth, we as humans will need more help than nature can supply. It's an undeniable fact because of the society we have created and we all live in.

Cancer is indiscriminate, it is relentless, it knows no boundaries, and it can be mortally dangerous. Cancer can even trick our own good cells into betraying their host—us. We as humans can't always fight those fights by ourselves. It does take a lot of nature, but it also takes dedicated physicians, it will take pharmaceutical companies, it takes medical advancements and technologies, and it takes getting down on our knees, praying and fighting the good fight of faith. Cancer may be a strong adversary, but it can be defeated, which means we should take full advantage of all the ammunition we have at our disposal. Plus, with all of the new medical advances our great minds are making, we are becoming more victorious over our enemy as each day passes.

Some of the medications I tried did make a difference—a small difference, yet still it was progress, and of course, some meds did not work for me. That's why there are so many elements out there for us guys to try. People are different, so one med may work great for some men and not for others. It may be the difference within the medications or it could be the human difference. Plus, it's not like you take one pill one day, and if it doesn't work, you try a different pill the next day and so on. The fact of the matter is I like to make notes and charts so I can see the difference, I had to let my body and my mind have at least an entire month with each different medication to become adjusted to the effects and make my notes in order that I could be sure of my findings. In the beginning, none of them worked immediately. The main thing about these meds, and something which I didn't care for, was one small fact—they all seemed to have small drawbacks or side effects. For instance, there was one med I tried which gave me headaches (not terrible migraine-type headaches. On the contrary, they were light or mild headaches, but they seemed to linger), and the strange thing about those headaches was they came not when I took the meds. No, it was like many hours later—sometimes the next day—is when I experience the side effects. At first, I didn't realize my headaches were from the meds because they came on me so much later. It was only after several weeks of trying the pill that I finally put one and one together to equal the headaches were being cause by the meds. You see, I only took the med once every six or seven days, and then, later on in the day, the headache would appear, and several times, it was the next day; however, over the length of many weeks, my super sharp Sherlock Holmes mind connected the two together.

Cialis was the medication that helped me the most overall, and surprisingly, it was also the first med which I was introduced to at the very start of the process. Plus, at the very start, I didn't have any ill side effects while taking them, but I believe it was because the starting medication was a very low dosage (5 mg). It wasn't 'til I took the higher mg dosage that the side effects came. Now I must say, when I did try the higher dosage meds, I only took them, like I said maybe once a week, and that's because most of the higher dosage mg meds are "as needed and only if you are sexually stimulated." Here's another Budd note: You need to understand that these meds don't give you an erection, your mind gives you an erection. The big job Cialis or any medication must accomplish is to help your body in pumping the necessary blood into the penis for your erection. In other words, your mind and body together must be sexually stimulated for the medication to work. Simply taking a Cialis and laying back in the recliner while watching the evening weather channel will not produce an erection. If that does happen, please send me an email with the news channel you're watching.

Now with Cialis, like all the other medication I used, I did experience a few side effects, and again, it was like twelve or more hours after ingesting; however, this time, it wasn't just the light, mild headaches (which I can't stand, because you can't get away from headaches no matter what you do. They're right there with you), this new side effect came in the form of lower back pain which, for me, is uncomfortable yet manageable. When the pain came, I could use my recliner or sofa to rest and take all the weight off my back which, in turn, would lower my discomfort level. The reason I reference Cialis more than other meds is simple and innocent. It happened to be the one med which, I noticed, gave me the best results while using it coupled with the least amount of side effects and nothing more than that. I honestly didn't write down or record the date during my rehab my doc started me on Cialis, and for that, I must apologize to you; however, it was quite early on, perhaps one month in, but I did record the dosage level of the medication I was introduced to in the very beginning, and it was only a 5 mg dosage, which happens to be a low amount, especially when I compared it to other meds on the market, which I have seen go up to twenty and to forty and may go as high as sixty. My personal advice is to start with this lower dosage and see if you are compatible with the medication and their side effects. All meds will have some side effects, and it never hurts to test the water before diving in.

For now, this is the way I understand how it all works. Since it's is such a low dosage, I was instructed to take one tablet each day and at the same time of day to treat erectile dysfunction, but that is not what I did. I like to study things first and then act on it. So I only took it once every three days. I was a little hesitant and playing it safe. After two weeks of no difference and no side effects, I proceeded with the proper instructions of one pill (5 mg) a day every day, and that's exactly what I did, and being truthful, after about eight days, there was a difference. Still, I only noticed a small difference, which goes back to me saying that, in my own personal situation, it probably would take me a longer time to improve anyway. I honestly think it was me, not the meds. When I say "me" and not the meds, I mean my blood vessels and the associated nerves that had to heal properly in order to work together properly. I think if my stuff would have worked together physically and I took some of the meds, I am sure things would have been quite different. Now, after many months and still working on my rehab, coupled with so little improvement, I was moved up to the 20 mg Cialis, and with this higher dosage, there was an improvement. Still, the improvement was not enough to penetrate (almost and that was interesting), and again, for me, it's going to take longer. Also for me, I really don't think there was anything that would give me a rock-hard erection at this particular time of my recovery. My insides had to heal (blood vessels and nerve endings), and the doc told me it would take time, maybe a long time, and in some males, it takes a year or possibly longer, as in my case. I was unfortunately one of the longer ones. Also, by this time in my journey, I have read such a multitude of informational material that I knew it takes a long time for some gentlemen, and I also knew that, for some men, unfortunately, it does not return. Believe me, I was praying hard that I was not in the group where it does not return. Now, for the 20 mg, I would only use this higher dosage when needed. I did not take it daily like the lower dosage. Just different viewpoints, I think, for different men. At this time, I would like to take a moment and give high praise to the makers of Cialis and, for that matter, all the other meds on the market today for helping males around the world to achieve the hardness needed to penetrate for the satisfaction of both partners. It is a wonderful thing. This can be a very difficult and heartfelt time for many gentlemen and their partners because of the ED difficulties and the problematic situations it carries with it. It's awkward to even speak about. So if you have never experienced any of this, you should be thanking God for your fine health.

Now, after saying all that, I will tell you a short story about the 20 mg dosage. This story happened to me about three years into my recovery process. I was cleaning out my dresser drawers and found an old three-pack of Cialis 20 mg tablets. Well, I haven't used any helper meds for well over a year—happy to say I didn't need them—but my chart making curiosity got the better of me, and I slipped one of the tablets out of the container pack and waited for a day when my wife and I would be going out for a night at the theater, a romantic dinner, and a romantic time at home to finish out our Friday night. I took the tablet about four in the afternoon, we were back home by eleven that evening, and wow, this time, hallelujah, brother, I really did hang a bath towel on it, which made me want to beat on my chest and jump around the room. Like I stated earlier, I recovered to about 95 percent, and this tablet just kicked in the other 5 percent and it made a difference, but I don't like taking medications, and it did come with a small backache. I really don't need the extra kick. I have recovered nicely and have been told I do quite well without it. However, it did show me that these medicines which are out there on the market for us men do work, and for some men and their spouses, these meds are a welcome additive and a blessing. In some cases, it takes a lot of hands-on work (penile rehab) to get the blood and nerves healed enough for the meds to kick it into overdrive.

There are a variety of different philosophies, ideas, medicines, pills, and devices on the open market to help us gentlemen with the seriousness of erectile dysfunction (ED) in both areas. First is attaining an erection, and second is also maintaining an erection. Both are important, and most of these medicines will do that. They will very a little in the amount of their dosages too—from weak to strong. But be careful and take caution with your selection. I also must interject to you this important fact: Any and all of the many different elements in the open market for us guys to try should be shown to your doctor and allow him to advise you on the health and safety for your own particular situation. In fact, checking with the doctor is a wise thing to do, because some of these meds can be dangerous if taken along with any other meds or type of nitrates or other interacting drugs. In this day and age, there are so many potential drug actions, reactions, and interactions which could be detrimental to your health and personal safety. Believe me, it's always advisable to seek out professional help and advice from the doctor who knows you and your passed health history and will be able to tell you if something you are wanting to take may have a bad reaction with another medication you might be already taking. You surely do not want to end up in the ER like the guy in the movie *Something's Gotta Give*. Another note of safety, and my personal advice, is to be sure any of the meds you are wanting to try are produced by a United-States-based company and filled at an accredited pharmacy, even if you acquire them online.

I did a bit of research and found out this interesting fact—male enhancement drug manufacturing is a multi-*billion* dollar a year business, which means there are some unscrupulous people who will try and pull some of that money down and into their pockets with a less than perfect U.S. regulated drug. They will do that at your expense, so be cautious with online orders where you can't find out what is really in those pills you are ingesting. Now, a word about the online items out there for us guys to use. I tried a few different ones available, and honestly, there were a handful of things I didn't even want to try. A friend of mine purchased some of his pills from an online site, and after a bit of inquiring from me with him about his items, I found out they arrive at his house through the mail—quite convenient—but they come from China. Now just speaking for myself and using my own opinion in this situation, I would advise against this sort of thing. That's just my own personal opinion and frame of mind on this subject. I'm not convinced that anyone would know for sure what they are placing inside their body when you purchase something like this from a company that is outside the United States and is not United States based and/or controlled.

Here's a cute little story about another one of my acquaintances who thought he would try one of the many ED helpers that are out there in the market place today. This helper he tried was a "penile injection service," where a medication is actually injection into the penis to produce an erection. Stand back, my friends, because this produces an erection whether you are ready for it or not. He told me the injection didn't hurt (I find that a little hard to believe) and also said it was fairly simple and took only a few minutes to complete, although he did say it was a little on the expensive side; he did not tell me how expensive nor did I ask. I believe he told me he signed up for a four-injection service which could be completed over many weeks or months if he liked. Well, he went in for his first service and received his first injection, and once the med was injected, it only took about five minutes and it began to stiffen, and after about fifteen minutes, he said it was hard—very hard. He was back at hanging a towel on it and even held his coat in front of him as he left the building. The service worked well beyond his expectations. Here's the funny part: After receiving his injection, as he stepped outside the medical building, he immediately got right on his cell phone, called his wife, and enlightened her on his situation. He told her she needed to leave work and come home as quick as she could. He told me it worked great and remained hard for three hours. Also, when it began to unstiffen, there was just a small bit of pain from being hard for such a long a time. I think we would all say that's understandable. He did say you have to be ready to use it because once it's injected, it's only minutes before the erection begins to take shape. He was told beforehand that these injections normally last two or three hours; however, there could be prolonged hardness and may last a little longer.

This worked quite well for him, but for me, this was one of those handful of items that I didn't want to try along with another device called the penis vacuum pump—which, some say, works very well, but I found out this is only short lived—and a strange item called the penis ring, which I didn't try but did investigate. It works on the theory of letting blood pass into the penis but limits it exit which, in turn, holds the blood inside which, in turn, produces a harder time. These items may all work and may be a great help to many men, and if it works for you, great! Go for it, partner, and be happy, but I guess I may be a little old fashioned, because honestly, I just wanted everything to work normally for me or, perhaps I should say, naturally for me (maybe it's my tree hugger mentality), but that's the way I am, so please don't look unfavorably on me. Fortunately, I will tell you that, for me, the penile rehab has worked out; it just took a long while, just a little over a year, but I would like to say it's working without the use of any exterior stimulus or devices, and I say amen to that.

Space for notes:

CHAPTER 9

Conclusion

Since you are obviously reading this book, I presume you are now traveling through a similar journey, or perhaps you just received the mind-bending news from the doctor that you have been diagnosed with cancer, that petrifying and frightening darkness that comes with the "C" word. If so, you are about to embark on this uncertain rollercoaster journey yourself. I'll give you the same advice I give other guys. It's important to know, in all this, you are not alone, and no one needs to go through this journey by themselves. If you search out others who have gone down this path, you'll find friends you haven't even met yet. Reaching out to others and speaking with other men who are now on the other side of their journey is a good thing. You will find many have tread down the same path you are now facing. This same path is now your future journey and must be met with optimism and forward thinking, not loneliness and despair. It will be for your own benefit to confront this situation with an optimistic outlook and mindset—to be a winner, to be a survivor. Again, I'll say use everything as a source of motivation. Once you start the process, you need to follow through with it in its entirety. Once it begins, you might as well jump tight in the saddle, wrap the rope around your hand, and ride it 'til the buzzer sounds.

Something that I found interesting was that most men who have gone down this road before us are ready to speak about their journey to you and to help calm your fears. When you first hear the "C" word and its ugly dark boney finger is directly pointed at you, your world will stop. Mine certainly did. Even your mind and breathing will seem to stop (mine also). Your world will change at that very moment in time. It will be frightening as your mind reels in disbelief. All of those horrific reactions and runaway emotions are entirely normal, and you want to know something; since they are normal and they do happen with regularity, perhaps we as humans need to go through them at times. Maybe we need to freak out and run around like chickens with their heads cut off so we can see plainly again with a broader perspective in our thoughts once we come back down to earth. For myself, my entire world changed in a New York second with only one short phone call right in the middle of a sunny day. When you experience these shocking moments, please take a step back. Take a little time to wrap your mind around what's happening. Let the news settle in. Believe me, this is some distressingly stressful news. It can frighten the life out of you, and it will surely frighten your family also, but you'll need to deal with it in your own way, but deal with it you must—and will.

I dealt with this dark time by keeping the dreadful news to myself for a few days. I needed to wrap my own mind around the situation and grieve in my own way. I had to grasp hold of my own personal circumstances before laying it out to my family, friends, and the rest of the universe to hear. Like other guys, I was asking myself question after question after question, and of course, since I was asking myself all these questions, I wasn't getting any helpful answers.

Four big questions that arose within my head were as follows:

1) How does one prepare himself to deal with such a thing let alone tell his wife and family this kind of news?
2) How can I prepare them to hear what I think might happen to me?
3) How will my wife react when I tell her that her soulmate might not be around to take care of her and that she might lose the love of her life?
4) What do I need to do quickly to help prepare my wife for her life ahead if I perhaps don't make it?

Something else I realized while I was asking myself all these questions; I didn't have a "last will and testament," which was one of the first things I accomplished. Also, since I've been healthy my entire life, I didn't even have a life insurance policy to pass on to my wife for the needed assistance to help her in the coming times in case I didn't make it through this. These thoughts and a few more were becoming a reality to me, and they were all unnerving and a bit chilling, and I realized, most of it was all due to my own procrastination in life. I also had other questions, which I'm quite sure other people have had, and the most famous one is "Why me, God?" What did I do in life to warrant this tragedy, and why has it befallen on my shoulders? Did I mess up somewhere in the game of life? Again, why me? I'm one of the good guys in life, I have a good family, I attended church, I've worked hard all my life and worked honestly for what I have, I pay my taxes, volunteer in the community. Why would this peril befall me?

Time for another quick story concerning the life of Budd, and I assure you, this story will help you appreciate where I was positioned on the ball field of life just moments before receiving the dreaded phone call. Better yet, instead of starting with the phone call, let's go back and start several years earlier than the call. We'll start with the liquidation of the family construction company and the selling of some property. At that point in time during my life, I really desired to slow down the speed I was traveling in my everyday life. You know, move out of the fast lane. I have driven in the fast lane for many, many years, and I figured I'd been speeding long enough. I gave my situation a lot of thought and believed the best way to accomplish this slow down process was to remove the items in my life that seemed to be occupying my waking hours—eighteen waking hours a day at times. Some weeks, especially with the construction company within the good warm summer months, it was work, work, work every day, including weekends. Being in the construction business in Colorado, you have a window of opportunity, and it comes in the form of good weather. Believe me, doing outdoor construction, it's essential to take full advantage of that warm weather window. In addition to running a construction business, I owned ten rental units. I also had a family, was on my neighbor HOA board, and adding a little more into the formula was some volunteer work I did. I was busy to say the least—too busy. If I truly wanted to change lanes and slow down, I had to change gears and pull my life into the slow lane. I knew all the time-occupying items had to be dealt with. So I made a chart and lined them up in order, starting at the easiest to rid myself of and then moving up toward the most difficult to eliminate. The first two items to go were also the easiest decisions to make. They were the HOA board position and volunteer work. They were simple to cancel, and if my life became too relaxed, they are easy to restart, which makes them easy decisions for the cut. Going up to the top of the chart, I came to the two hardest decisions to make, which were also the largest time-consuming items on the list. These two were the construction company business, which had been in existence for over sixty years, and the townhome rental units.

My grandfather started the construction company in the 1940s and worked it well. After many years, he pulled my father into it. My father naturally continued it side by side with his father. As with all things, time passed, and my grandfather retired. My father was now in full control and continued the business by himself. After many more years, my father pulled me into it, so naturally, it was my turn to work side by side with my father, which I did, and we worked the business together along with my mother. When it was time for my father to retire, I naturally continued it by myself; however, the story ends there, for it saddens me to say, unlike my father and his father, "I didn't have a son to pull into it." Plus, the thought of selling it was out of the question. The reason was simple: That business and the company's name, "Nielsen Plastering Inc.," worked on thousands of buildings in the state and established an excellent and reputable record of completed jobs in Colorado. Over the years, "Nielsen Plastering Inc.," established a fine and honorable reputation with the "Associated General Contractors of America," known as the AGC of Colorado. Nielsen Plastering Inc. was known as the gold standard of our specification section in the construction community (no brag, just fact). So the thought of handing the gearshift over to someone else who might tarnish our family name with less than honorable work was not acceptable. So the decision I made was to auction off the workings, close out the books, and retire the name. It was not an easy decision to make because of the family history connected with it and its size. However, it was one decision that had to be made if I really desired to reach my new life goals, and I honestly did want to reach them. Also, within my elimination list was to rid myself of the most time-consuming and difficult rental properties we owned and managed. These were all difficult decisions; nevertheless, they were decisions I were willing to make if it allowed my wife and myself to create a life together rather than just existing together in life. We both realized we needed to make some difficult and important changes if we wanted to spend more quality time with each other before it was too late, and believe me, my friend, when I say an unforeseen and totally unwanted cancer diagnosis will surely make everything too late.

When all the before-mentioned time-consuming factors in my life were all together and running at high RPMs, I was a busy man, too busy for my own good and too busy for my own health. For what seemed like countless years, my alarm clock started my day at 4:44 a.m. Even during daylight savings time, I was still up before the sun. By 6:00 a.m., I was not only up and dressed, but I was already out the front door and headed for the office. At the end of the day, when I arrived home from work, my wife and I would spend a couple of precious hours with each other. After that precious but too little time with her, I was off to bed because of the early hour I needed to awake and run the human rat race the following day, continuing the repetitive process once more. Seriously, my life was like the movie *Groundhog Day*, only without all the funny stuff. Those couple of hours (and sometimes it wasn't even a couple of hours) my wife and I spent together in the evening were nice, and thank God for them, but they weren't the quality time nor the quantity of time we needed; life was going by fast. So I made some difficult decisions and started to change things which, in turn, would allow me to move my life vehicle into the slower and less complicated lanes on the highway of life, but of course, that's not as easily accomplished as it may sound. After making many small cuts on my list, it was time to make the decision on the construction company. I didn't have a son who could continue the business, and honestly, I was tired too and wanted to retire. I was standing ready to lead our family construction business up into the north forty pastures and let it retire in the shade right along with myself.

It took a year and half of getting my ducks in a row, such as winding up the already-in-place contracts the construction company was obligated to complete, before I could begin the liquidation process of the company. I contacted a quality auctioneer company, and it took two and a half weeks to collect, clean, palletize, and label all the equipment for the upcoming auction. I've got to say, it's a two-sided situation to put oneself into. On one hand, I was glad to be done with all the never-ending and burdensome responsibilities like the OHSA regulations, the everyday architect and engineering hassles, the always-present employee problems (which, I swear, sometimes it was like operating an adult day care), and all the insurance problems, dealing with attorneys, and the multitude of other miscellaneous time-consuming items that surround a person who is involved in running a corporation. Now on the other hand, which is the much brighter side of this story, it was such a relief, like literally having a heavy weight lifted off your shoulders, because you know your life is about to get easier and personal time is about to get better too. However, out of the hundreds of pieces of equipment and the associated gear, all the hand tools, dump trucks, loaders, pickups, office equipment, computers, file cabinets, and miscellaneous items which had to go, during the auction, there were three particular items which I predominantly remember, and these three pieces really wounded my spirit but also touched my heart as I watched them being loaded onto another companies' trailer by people I have never met and hauled down the street, never to be seen by me again, and all right in front of my eyes. One of the precious three items was a bright safety yellow-painted, front-tilt forklift which my father purchased when I was a little kid and would give me rides on. As I got older, he also taught me to operate it. Our company used that forklift expressly in the two warehouses; it never left the property its whole life. The second item was the large black walnut desk where my mother sat and performed her job for what seemed, to me, like a hundred years, and the last item to go was the old soda pop machine; it only took quarters nothing else, and it was one quarter to purchase one can of soda pop. Honestly, when those three items got loaded up (and those three were, out of the multitude of pieces, the last to leave), I had tears in my eyes.

It took another year and a half after I auctioned off the construction company before I was in a place where I acted on the final decision, which was to sell the time-consuming rental town home units. The rental units were not as difficult to rid myself of like the construction company was, because unlike the company, they did not pull on my heart strings; they were only ledger entries in my computer Excel charts. Fortunately, I found a broker who found a client who stepped up to the plate and purchased all the units in one large real estate deal. It was the best way to sell them too—all at once. After the rentals were out of my life, I wanted to shout from the rooftops because my life really changed, and I would like to say it was a change for the better; life seemed to get brighter. I had more time for my wife and my life instead of spending my life behind a desk or on the road in a pickup truck with one hand on the gearshift while the other hand was holding a phone to my ear. Oddly enough, as time marched on, I really enjoyed my newfound freedom. I found myself taking care of the house, preparing dinners for my wife, and throwing a stick in the park for my new little pal, Parker, a little black-and-white Sheltie sheepdog whose main goals in life were to play, have fun in the sun, run around, and take a nap in the grass under a shade tree, and somehow, he began teaching me his beliefs. Believe it when I say my days were pleasurable. I had time for life or just time to work in the backyard, and I had some money in my pocket. It was incredible, it was enjoyable, and I was having fun doing what I wanted to do instead of doing what I had to do; a small difference when you read those words, but a huge difference in the reality of those words.

After auctioning off the construction company and later selling most of the rental properties, life just continued to get better. My wife received a promotion at her job, and we were happy in our newfound lives together. One more pristine year passed by, and our realtor finally located that one special ranch-style home we had been searching for; we secured it and moved into our beautiful new house. Life was moving in the right direction, and this is the cherry on top of Budd's banana split. Fortunately, I was able to retire at an early age. All the little pieces of Budd's life puzzle were finally coming together, and the picture was looking pretty rad. Really, dude, I'm telling you, I was perfectly set up to enjoy a nice relaxing life taking care of my wife, our new home, and my little pal Parker.

The best gift of all? Now I'm ready to appreciate life and live it with the woman I seem to be falling in love with all over again, and she's the woman I consider to be the perfect companion for me. So in summary, I was in a place where most guys would say, "That dude's sitting pretty." Because we planned for our future and we diligently saved our money, my wife and I achieved a plateau where we could begin to take life a little calmer, enjoy life as a couple, and not have to worry so much. The "not worry so much" part is unbelievably price-less. Needless to say, our life was looking up. I had the cruise control locked on, the windows were rolled down, and the radio cranked. All things looked like smooth sailing from here on out. I was loving it and she was loving it too. However, on the far distant future horizon, there was a black cloud building, and no one had seen it coming; it was that dreaded phone call, and when it arrived, all hell broke loose. It popped the proverbial bubble. Well, to be more precise, it didn't pop; it exploded.

As dark as it seemed to me, during that moment of time, and as dark as it may seem to you right now in yours, you have to keep moving and looking forward. Think of it this way—you're inside of a long, narrow, and poorly-lit tunnel and you can't see much of anything. So naturally, it's difficult to know where to start or even what you should do. You are kind of stuck in one place. But I can help. When you're in this darkness and confused about what to do, stick out your arm and keep reaching 'til your hand touches against the tunnel's side wall. Touch the wall and gather some information about it, get your bearings, so to speak, and then, against all odds, you begin slowly trudging forward because you see there is a small light at the end of this tunnel. OK, that's just a metaphor, but here's what I'm really saying—reach out for help and get all the information about your tunnel (your situation, get the goods on the cancer), find out all you can about it, research the internet, google it, ask the doctors, talk to the people around you, and read the books because you need all that information in your head in order for you to make an educated and well-informed decision concerning where you are at and what's confronting you, and then you can confidently combat it and move forward not backward, looking up, not down. One of Stephen Hawking's most famous quotes is "Look up toward the stars, not down at your feet." Make your decisions based on educated information, not guesswork. How many times have you made a hasty choice only to have it turn bad or back fire in your face? Don't do that here, my friend. The enemy is too great.

Thankfully, medical technology advances every day, and I pray it just keeps going upward and keeps getting better, more improved, and faster for the benefit of us all. The ideas and new techniques the hospitals and medical professionals perform in today's world are all quite amazing, and the people are downright remarkable, educated, and dedicated to their profession, their true craft, and the wonderful work they perform. The good news is that things will continue to get brighter with every advancement. It may seem bleak and unbearable to you at this moment; it certainly seemed bleak to me in my moment. In fact, that bleak phone call I received on that sunny day had me truly believing I was given a death sentence (can't get much bleaker than that), and I'm telling you here and now, I naturally sank really low. But take heed, my brother, and be certain of this: I went through the darkness, others have gone through the darkness, and you too can make it through this darkness. Others went through the unknowing, the sadness that any cancer diagnoses can bring, all the uncertainty in addition to the multitudes of difficult decisions which will have to be made, but the other gentlemen made their decisions, I made my decisions, and read my lips, "So will you." Believe me, I know what it feels like to have cancer in your body, and I won't sugarcoat it. I'll tell you straight up, it's not fun, it's not easy, and it can seem quite difficult and overwhelming at times. You are going to be devastated from the news, your world will begin to change, you are going to feel like you're isolated, and it seems as through the rest of the world will carry on its merry way and is oblivious to your problem and your sadness.

It's also time consuming to do all the research. I spent untold hours searching the web and reading different information. Beside all the decisions to make, you're also going to trust and rely on different people and on different doctors and hospital staff you don't even know and you've never met before. However, they are here to help you in this journey. Take confidence in these words: Those doctors and nurses, "they really do care." You'll need to rely on the information and knowledge of others to help make some tough medical decisions which are going to affect your life now and in your future as well as your family's life. Your heart will beat faster than you've ever felt before. Your mind will go through some changes too. Other gentlemen before us have gone through this dark time, and many have faced tougher times than us and tougher decisions than us due to the fact that some of the medical advances were not available to them at their time of crisis. This next thought might sound weird, but we should consider ourselves lucky because of the many options and solutions that are on our side and exist for us today. Doctors are continuously gaining more knowledge on these matters and refining the process. Many have gone through this tunnel before you and I, and many will journey through it after us. Speak with others who have gone through this, reach out to groups, even speak with your friends; they may know someone who has journeyed through this. The gentlemen I spoke with said they also felt dejected, alone, and disheartened at the beginning of their journey. It's only normal to have those feelings, so go ahead and have those feelings; fall down and cry if you want. I did.

But then, do this also: Keep your head up, keep your eyes facing forward, and keep telling yourself, "I'm going to make it." In fact, you should write that sentence down on some paper in your own handwriting and tape it to the front of the refrigerator. Have some faith in yourself and in your own strength, my brother. Think about this: No matter what avenue you chose to fight against this monster that is attacking you, and after you reach the light at the end of your tunnel and you have beaten this ugly monster, you'll be able to share your journey, your experiences, all your tips and your knowledge with others, and they will call you a survivor. The men I spoke with were frightened just like me, but they carried on, and a few of those guys didn't have a helper by their side. Since I said, "I was speaking with them," means they are alive and well and came out into the light at the end of their own dark tunnel. The majority of the guys were four to five years out of their ordeal and now felt that they had regained their life. Hope is out there for all of us.

I am currently around 95 percent in my recovery process. However, I'm not too sure after any type of cancer diagnosis and/ or cancer surgery that a person will be back to 100 percent of their presurgery normal life. One may never be what they were before such a life-changing occurrence, and that's because it is "life changing." Believe me, brother, both your physical state, and most definitely your mental state, have been altered. Now you can use this altered state for the betterment of yourself and your family.

Any cancer diagnosis is scary. It can also be a long and frightening ordeal. Find the strength to endure and plow through it, because then, you will be known as a *survivor*, and that word is big. You can share your story of hope and survival with others for the benefit of all; you can be an example for other guys.

Dude, I hope this information helped you. I will pray for your success and health.

Budd Nielsen

About the Author

Budd Nielsen was born and raised in Denver, as was his parents, which makes him a second-generation native Coloradoan. He began working at his family's construction company at a very young age. He became a certified welder and certified lather, and he completed various apprentice programs within the construction industry. He eventually ended up owning and operating the construction company which he was a part of for over forty years. He continues to share his story with those affected by any cancer diagnosis and all test and trials of treatment and recovery of prostate cancer. Budd and his wife still live in Colorado

www.ingramcontent.com/pod-product-compliance
Lightning Source LLC
Chambersburg PA
CBHW061401280526
45784CB00001B/330